## THE ULTIMATE GUIDE TO
## NATURAL BODY DETOXIFICATION

# DETOX YOGA

### SUWANREE AMESBUTR VELLA

Despite all the care taken in writing this book, an error may have slipped in. The author declines all responsibility concerning the practice of the exercises being presented. This book cannot replace a doctor or substitute for a medical treatment. It is up to the reader to take responsibility for safety and knowledge of self physical condition; the author cannot be held responsible for the consequences resulting from the use of this book.



First edition, September 2022.

**ISBN 979-8-3527-8270-5**

Suwanree Amesbutr Vella
www.amber-yoga.com

"Good health is not something we can buy. However, it can be an extremely valuable savings account."

Anne Wilson Schaef

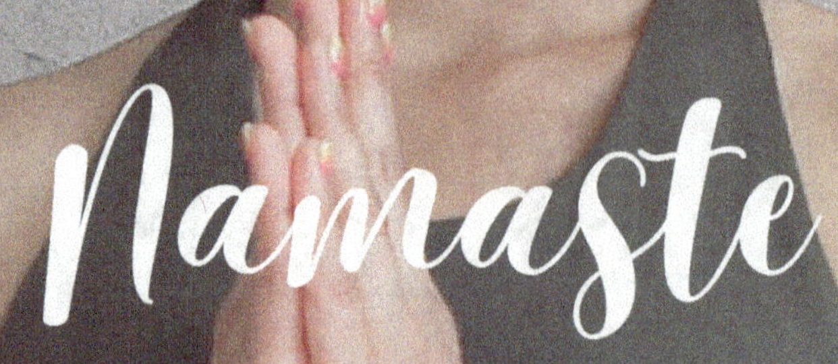
Namaste

# Contents

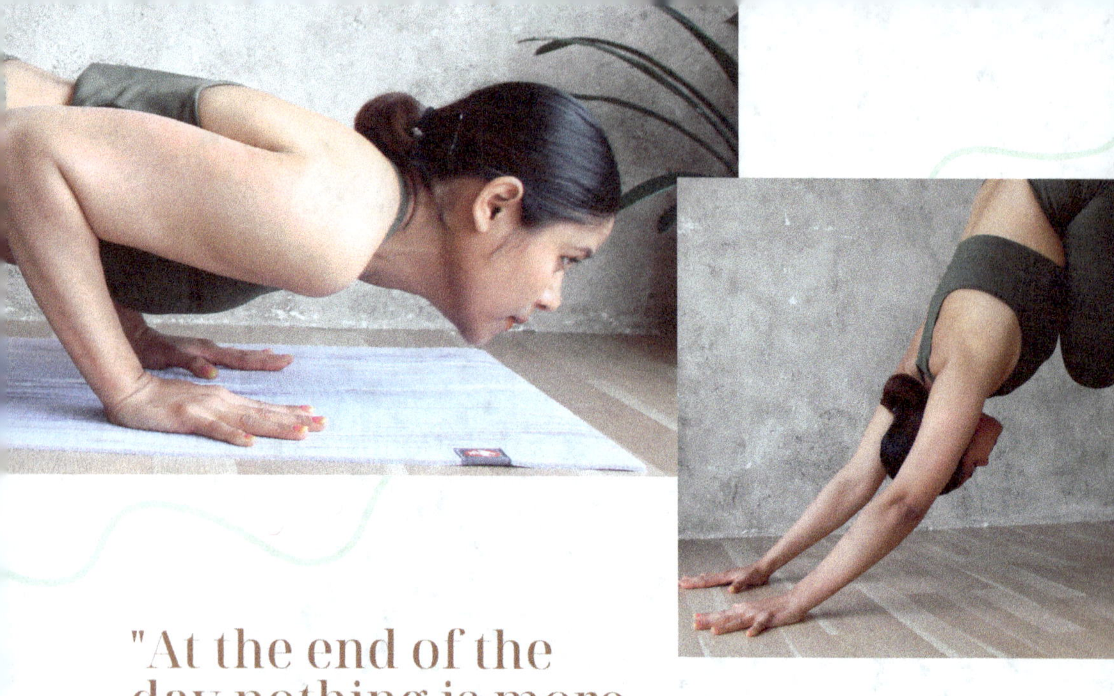

# "At the end of the day nothing is more important than having a good health."

I put myself in a stressful environment where I have ruined my own health for more than 10 years until I joined my first yoga class. I fell in love with how challenging the session was and the feeling after the session. I was impressed by the benefits of yoga and what our body is capable of. The more I practiced the more I realised that at the end of the day nothing is more important than having a good health.

I believe that our body is similar to a vehicle we must maintain attentively in order to move forward. Detoxification is another way to keep your body in good health. In this book you will learn how to self-detox naturally through breathing and practicing yoga, and improving your drinking, eating, and sleeping habits.

- SUWANREE A. VELLA

# What is Detoxification?

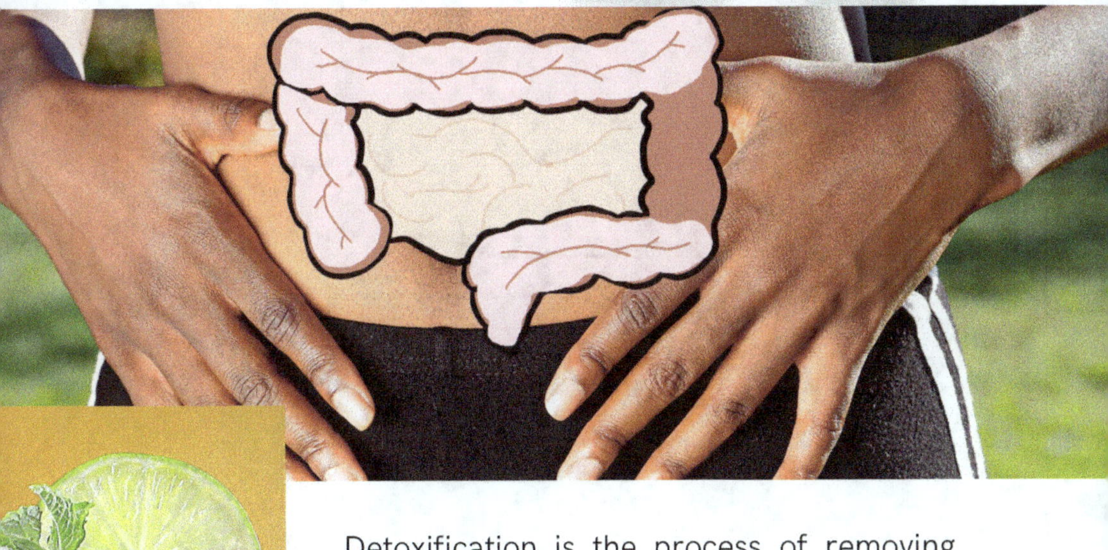

Detoxification is the process of removing toxic substances and the body detoxification is the process of removing toxin from the body. In the modern life we are exposed to significant amounts of toxin in food, water, air, cosmetics, and cleaning products to name a few.

To maintain a good health we might need to help our body to detoxify even though it is able to detoxify itself. An easy way to do so is to keep the detoxification organs - liver, kidney, digestive system, skin, and lungs - in good health. Efficient body detoxification helps improve the intestinal health and therefore prevents from various intestinal diseases.

# Intestinal health

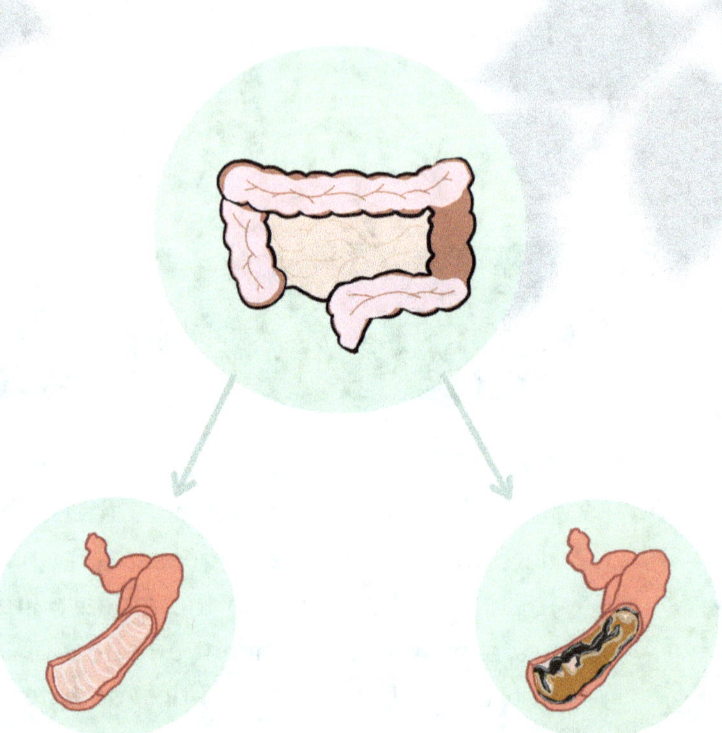

## Healthy Gut

- Looks clean and clear.
- No mucus and grease stains.
- Absorbs nutrients well.
- Feels full quickly.

## Unhealthy Gut

- There are mucus and grease stains.
- Dirty and smell (causing bad breath).
- Absorbs 2-3 times less nutrients.
- Feels full slowly (cause of obesity).

# Unhealthy Gut & Diseases

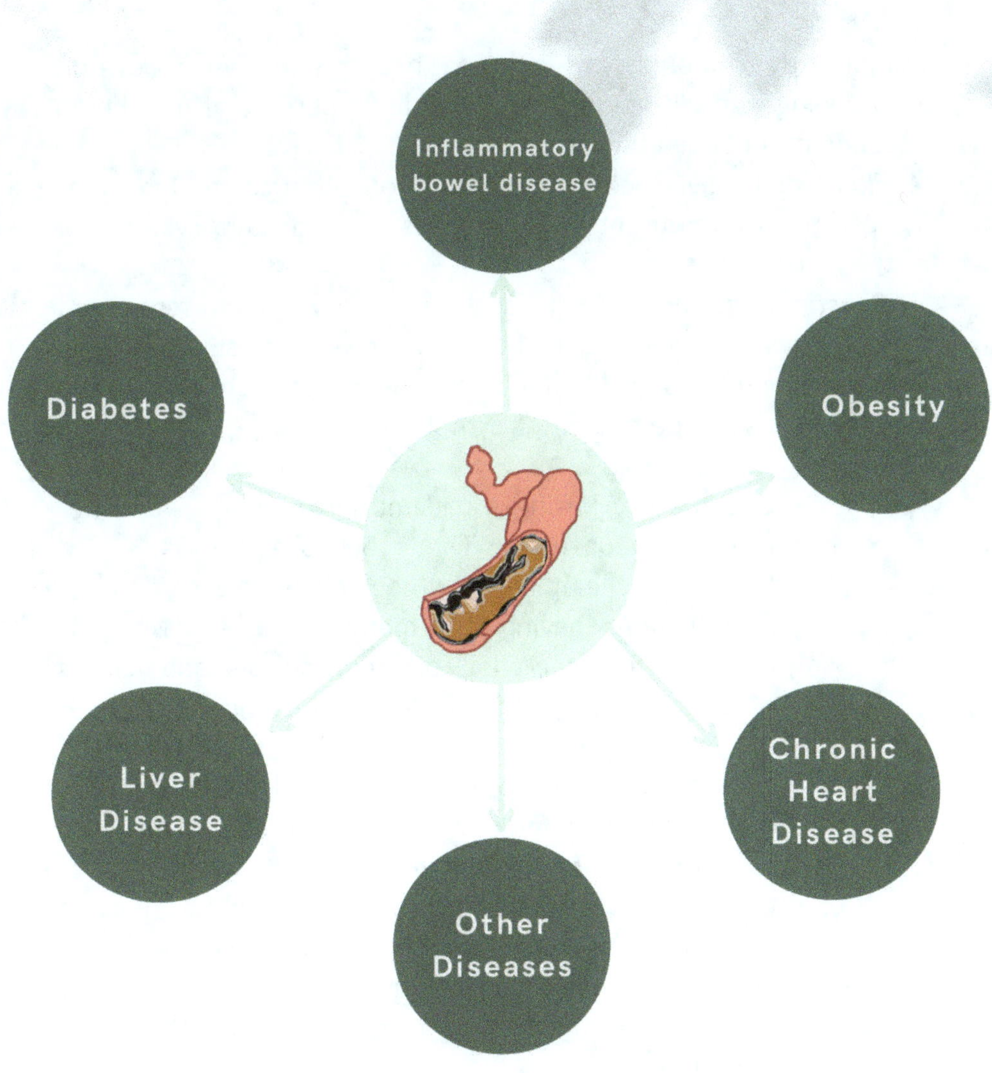

# Signs of an Unhealthy Gut

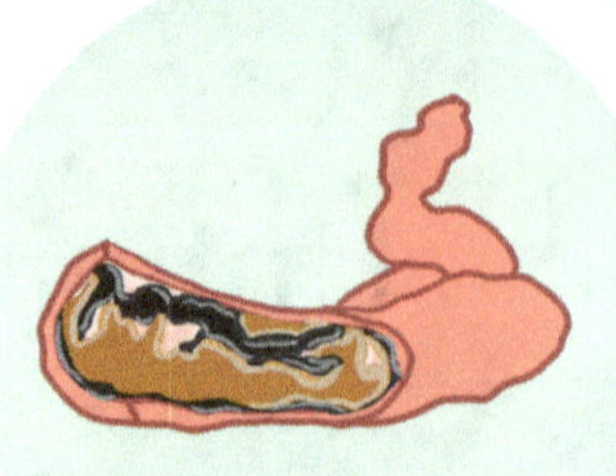

A simple way to monitor the intestinal health is to keep an eye on the following signs. If any of these symptoms persists, it may be an indication of an unhealthy gut.

- *Flatulence:* having colic and indigestion because the intestines absorb fewer nutrients which makes the digestive system not work properly.
- *Constipation:* certain toxins such as preservatives in fermented foods destroy the lining of the stomach and intestines causing the excretory system to malfunction. Not defecating for more than 3 days can be one of the symptoms.

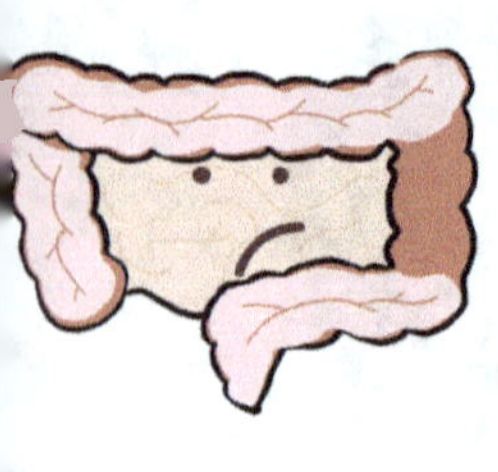

- *Bad breath:* having a bad morning breath even after brushing your teeth. That's because the waste and toxins that pile up have not been eliminated.
- *Rough skin:* having too many toxins in the body increases the secretion of free radicals and causes rough skin, acne, and wrinkles making one look older.
- *Insomnia:* the majority of your body's serotonin, which affects mood and sleep, is produced in the gut. So, when there's bacteria or inflammation in the gut, your sleep may be affected as well.
- *Unintentional weight gain:* when your gut is imbalanced, your body may struggle to absorb nutrients, store fat, and regulate blood sugar. Gaining weight may be caused by bacteria overgrowth or lack of nutrients.

# POOP

Poop colours can also give away the health situation of your gut.

## I am Yellow

Yellow to orange shade can be a sign of an intestinal infection, particularly if you also have diarrhea, fever, flu-like symptoms, or stomach cramps or if you eat a lot of yellow food.

## I am Brown

Brown poop is a healthy poop, no need for you to be warned, unless it is dark brown and difficult to pass.

## I am Green

Green hues can be caused by eating lots of leafy vegetables. In women, green poop may occur at certain times during pregnancy.

## I am Black

Black and dark brown poop, with or without blood, is not normal. It can imply that you have unhealthy gut.

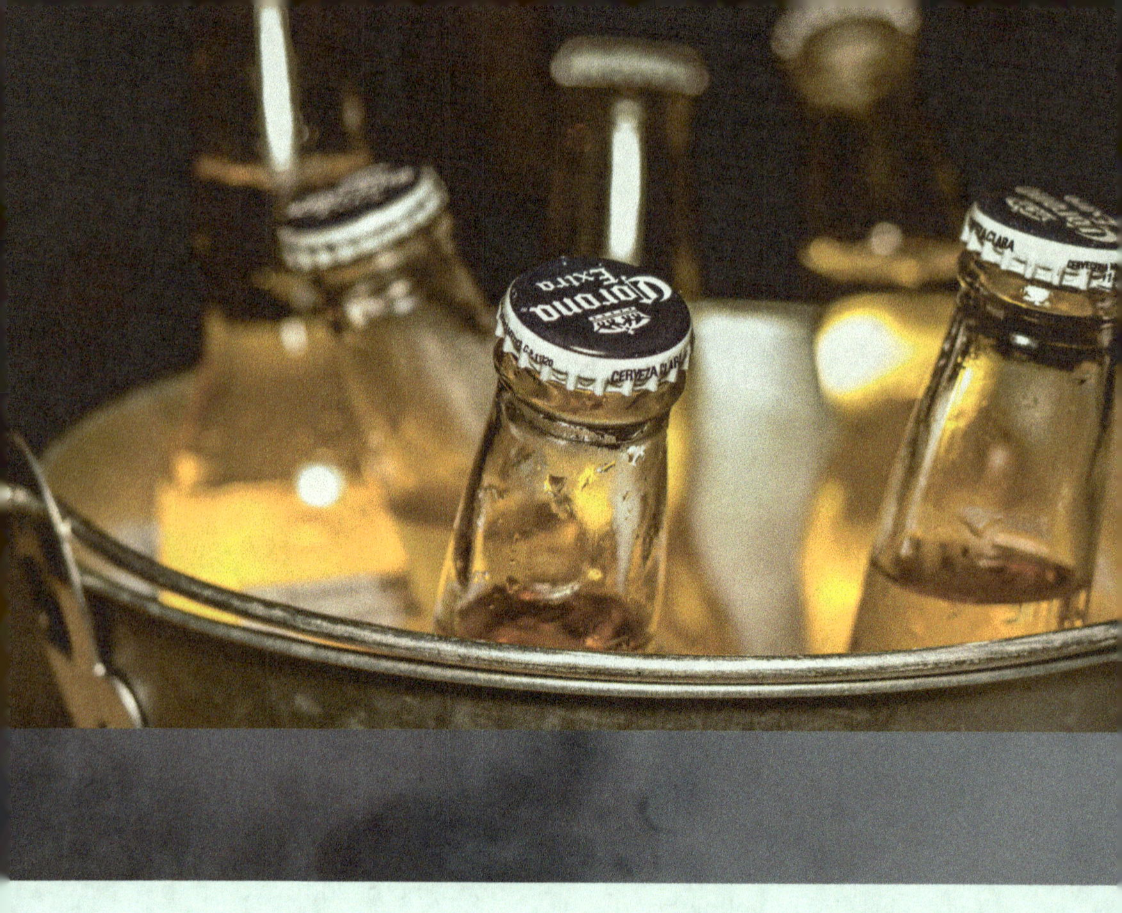

# Terrible Foods for your Gut

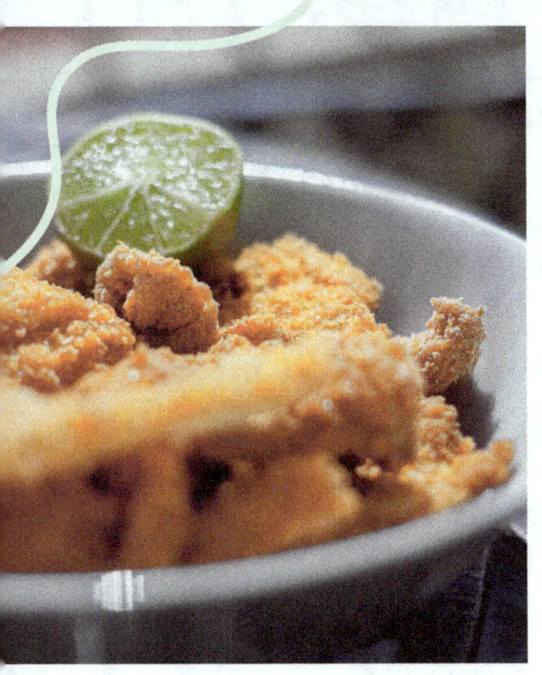

# 1. Fried Food

Fried food is more difficult to digest than fresh fruits and vegetables because it contains a lot of saturated and trans fats, and can lead to diarrhea, flatulence, and stomach pain.

# 2. Artificial Sweetener

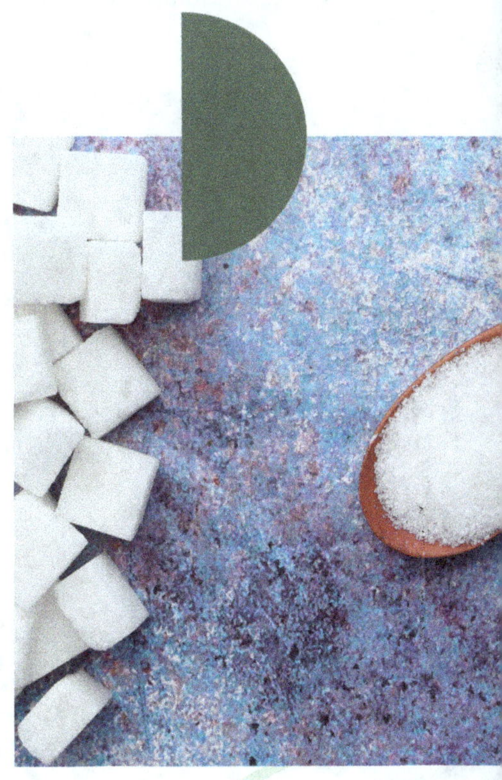

Artificial sweeteners can negatively affect the gut because of an increase of bacteria in the Bacteroids genus and a decrease of the Clostridiales genus.

A research published in April 2021 in the *International Journal of Molecular Sciences* suggests that some artificial sweeteners may be associated with the secretion of two harmful gut bacterias; E.coli and E. faecalis.

### 3. Alcoholic beverages

Drinking too much alcohol can harm your gut microbiome.

A research published in the journal *Gut Microbes in 2020* suggests that drinking alcohol excessively is associated with dysbiosis, which occurs when the bacteria in your gastrointestinal tract – including your intestines – become unbalanced.

### 4. Red meat

Red meats contain an abundance of L-carnitine which alters the bacteria in your gut. This can increase your risk of heart attack or stroke.

Higher red meat intake is also associated with an increased risk of colorectal cancer and inflammatory bowel disease.

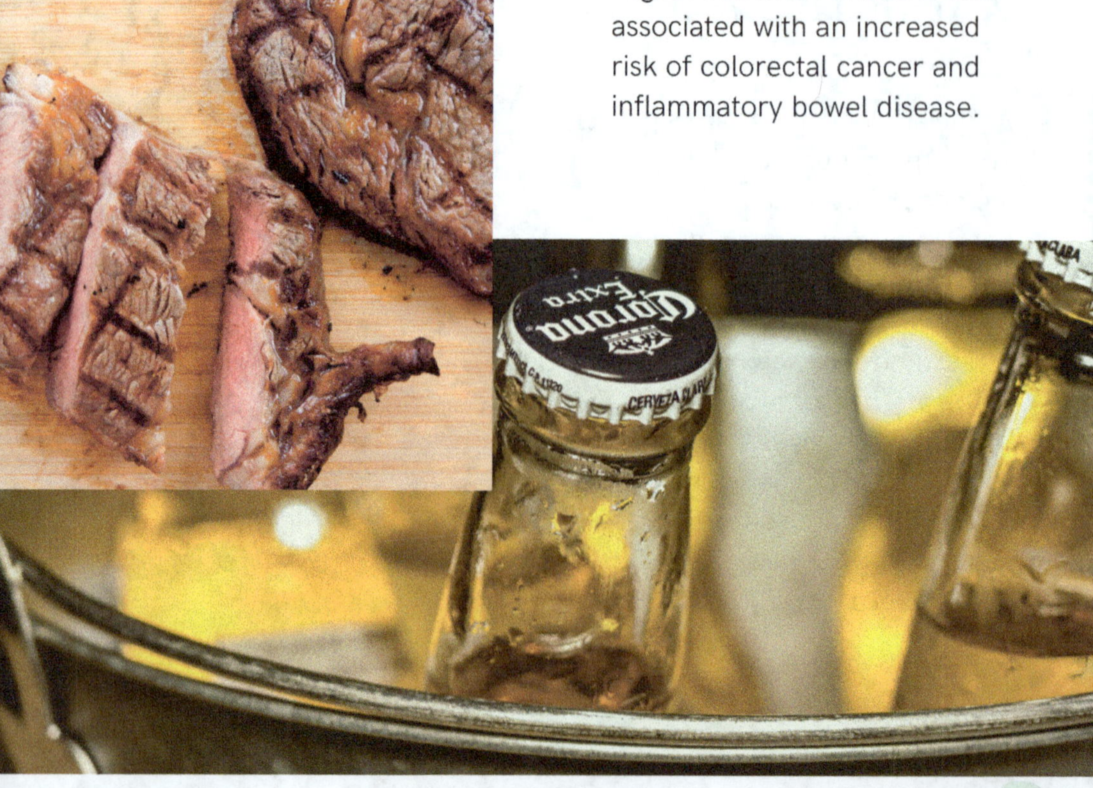

# 5. Processed foods

Processed foods such as bacon, ham, paté and sausage, canned vegetables, cakes, cookies, ready meals, contain additives and unhealthy amount of salt that can damage your gut microbiome.

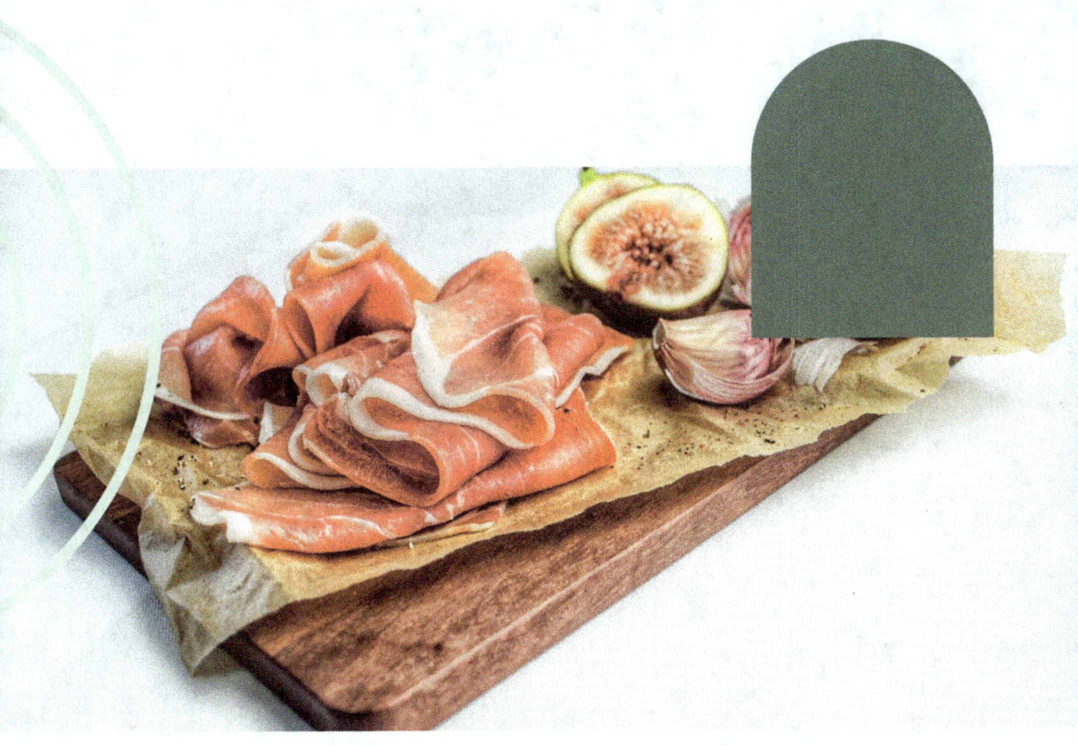

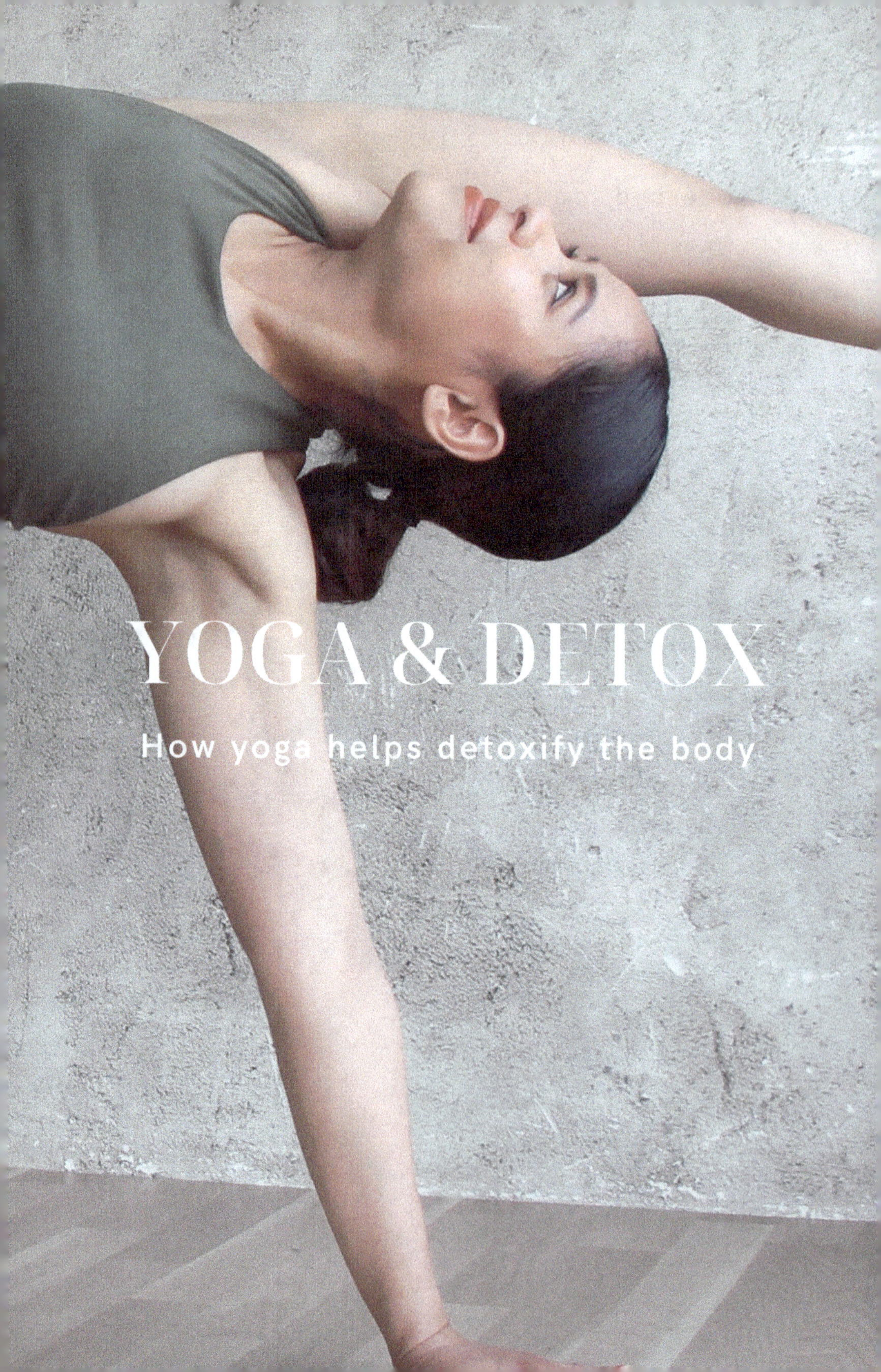

# YOGA & DETOX

How yoga helps detoxify the body

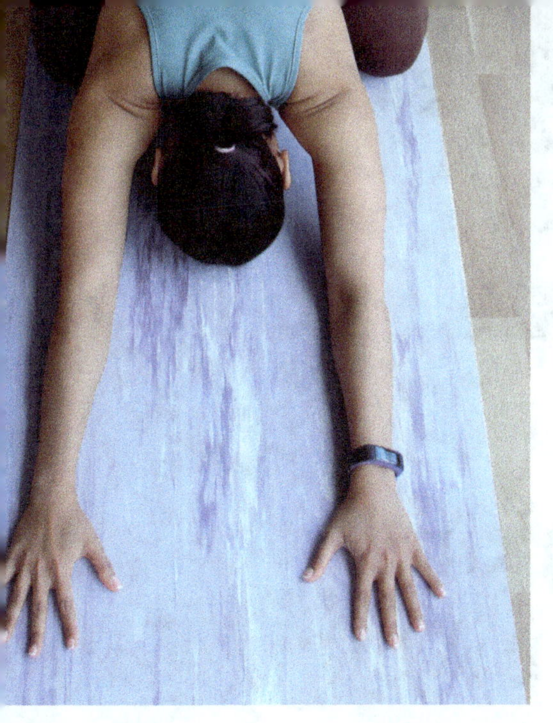

# Can Yoga Really Detox Your Body?

Our bodies have a built-in toxin removing system through liver, skin, kidneys, intestines, lymph nodes, and blood vessels and we easily get rid of toxin in the form of breath, urine, feces, and sweat.

Yoga provides tons of benefits and one of those is to detoxify the body on a physical, emotional and spiritual level.

Yoga poses such as twists, backbends, forward bends, and inversions, and yoga breathing techniques boost up the metabolism and aid toxin elimination.

Along with practicing yoga regularly, drinking enough water, getting enough sleep, maintaining a healthy diet will improve your metabolism and help your body to detoxify even better during the detoxification programme.

**DRINK ENOUGH WATER, HAVE ENOUGH SLEEP, MAINTAIN A HEALTHY DIET AND PRACTICE YOGA**

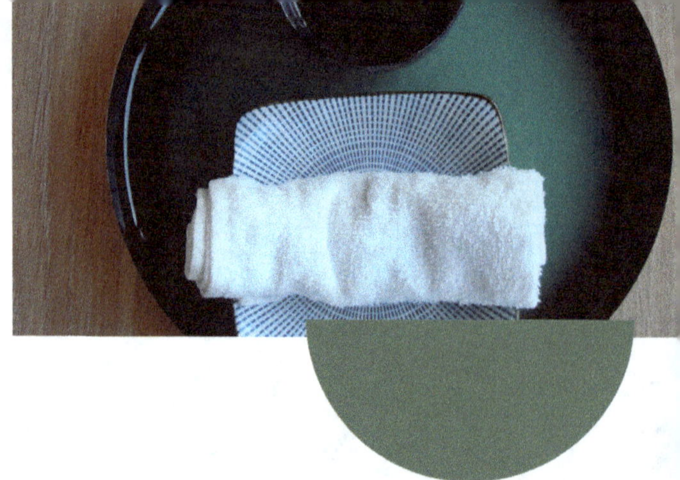

# Drinking Enough Water

60% of our body weight is made up of water. The human body, therefore, needs the right amount of water every day to maintain its balance and to use it in various bodily functions.  Each of us requires different amount of water per day depending on individual's physical condition and daily activities.

To know the exact amount of water you should drink per day you can use the following formula.

$$\frac{\text{Your body weight (kg) x 2.2 X 30}}{2}$$

= The amount of water you should drink

i.e.  your body weight is 60kg

$$\frac{60 \times 2.2 \times 30}{2} = 1{,}980 \text{ ml}$$

# Sleeping Better

### Get Enough Sleep

Getting a healthy amount of sleep is a key part of a good sleep pattern. Adults age 29-64 should sleep between 7-9 hours per night.

### Monitor Caffeine Intake

Caffeinated drinks, including coffee, tea, chocolate, and sodas, are among the most popular beverages in the world. Some people are tempted to use the jolt of energy from caffeine to try to overcome daytime sleepiness, but that approach isn't sustainable and can cause long-term sleep deprivation. To avoid this, keep an eye on your caffeine intake and stop consuming it at least 6 hours before bed.

### Be Mindful of Alcohol

Alcohol affects the brain in ways that can lower sleep quality, and for that reason, it's best to avoid alcohol in the lead-up to bedtime or at least 4 hours before bed.

### Bedtime Routine

It is almost impossible for your body to get accustomed to a healthy sleep routine if you're constantly waking up at different times. Pick a wake-up time and stick with it, even on weekends or other days when you would otherwise be tempted to sleep in.

### Switched Off

Tablets, smart phones, and laptops can keep your brain wired, making it hard to truly wind down. The light from these devices can also suppress your natural production of melatonin.

As much as possible, try to disconnect for 30 minutes or more before going to bed.

### Avoid Heavy Meals

Having a heavy meal less than 4 hours before bed can make it harder to fall asleep as your body is still digesting.

# DETOX YOGA POSES

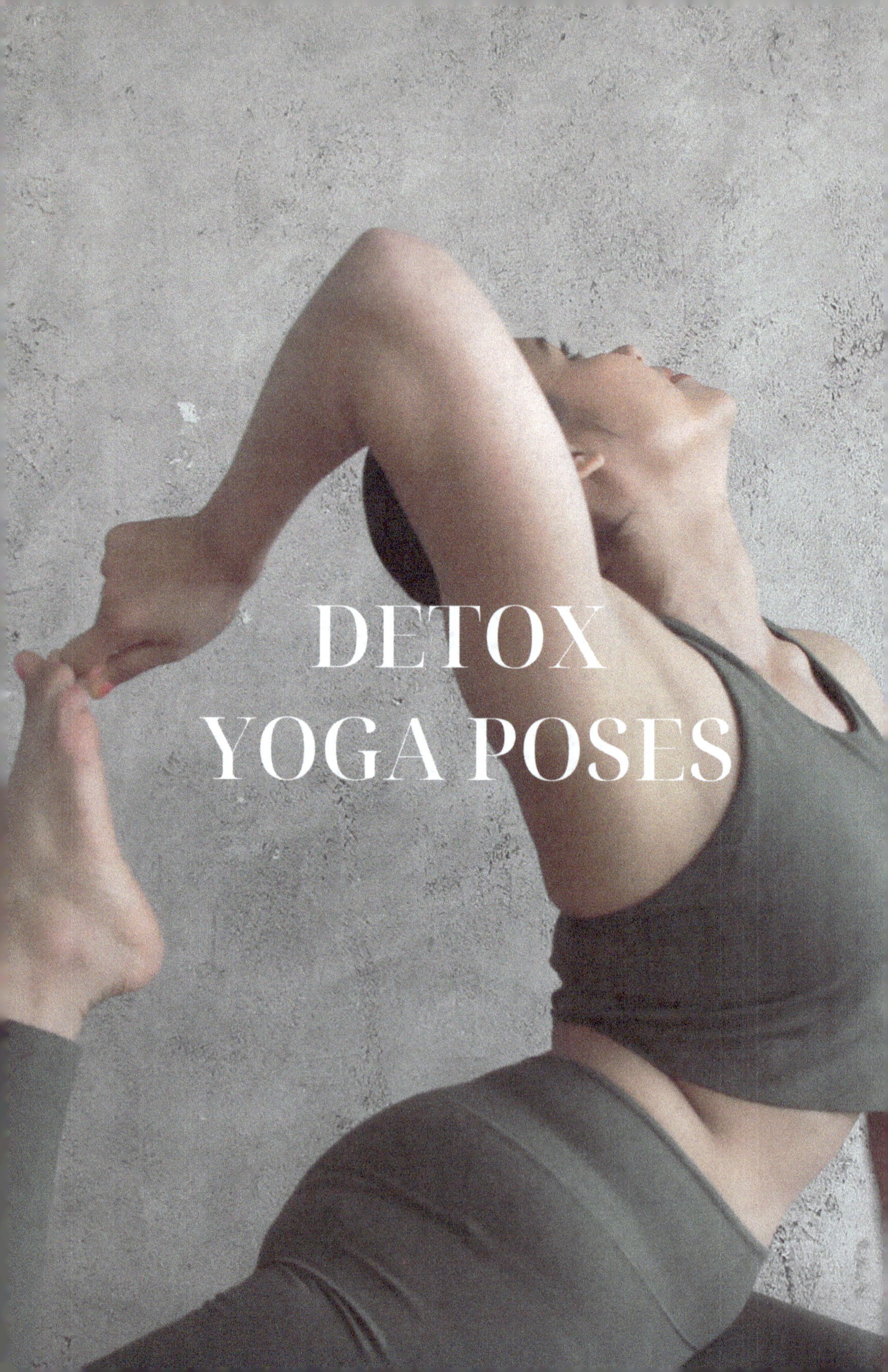

# Detoxification
# Yoga Poses

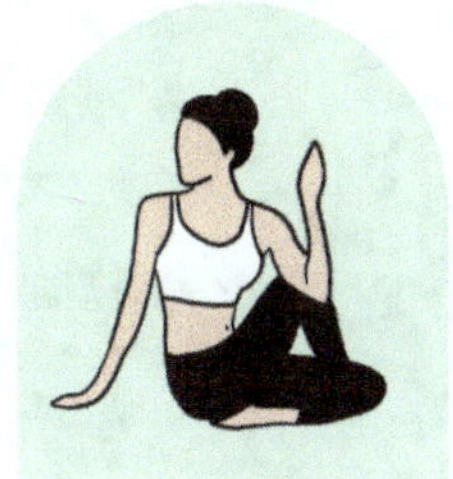

## TWISTS

Twisting poses stimulate the blood flow to the liver, gall bladder, stomach, spleen and intestines, and effectively help detox your body.

## BACKBENDS

Back-bending poses encourage digestion and aid elimination of waste in your body by applying gentle pressure to the abdomen.

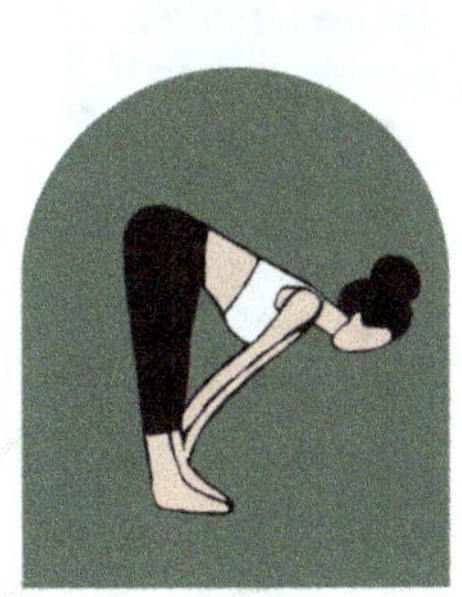

## FORWARD BENDS

The compress at the belly while practicing forward bend poses helps stimulate digestion and aid toxin elimination.

## INVERSIONS

Inversions poses help improve the immune system, stimulate your thyroid gland and boost your metabolism.

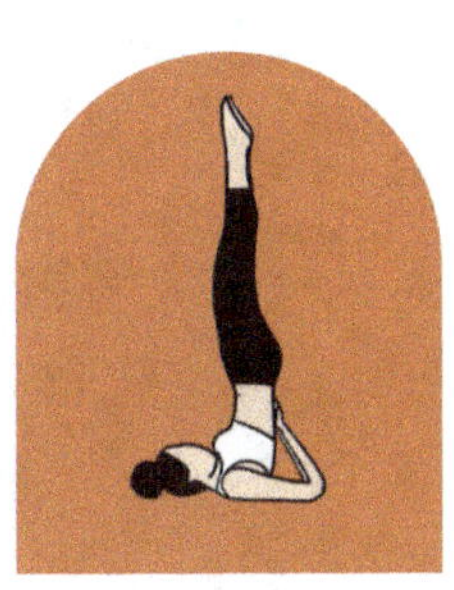

# Revolved Chair Pose

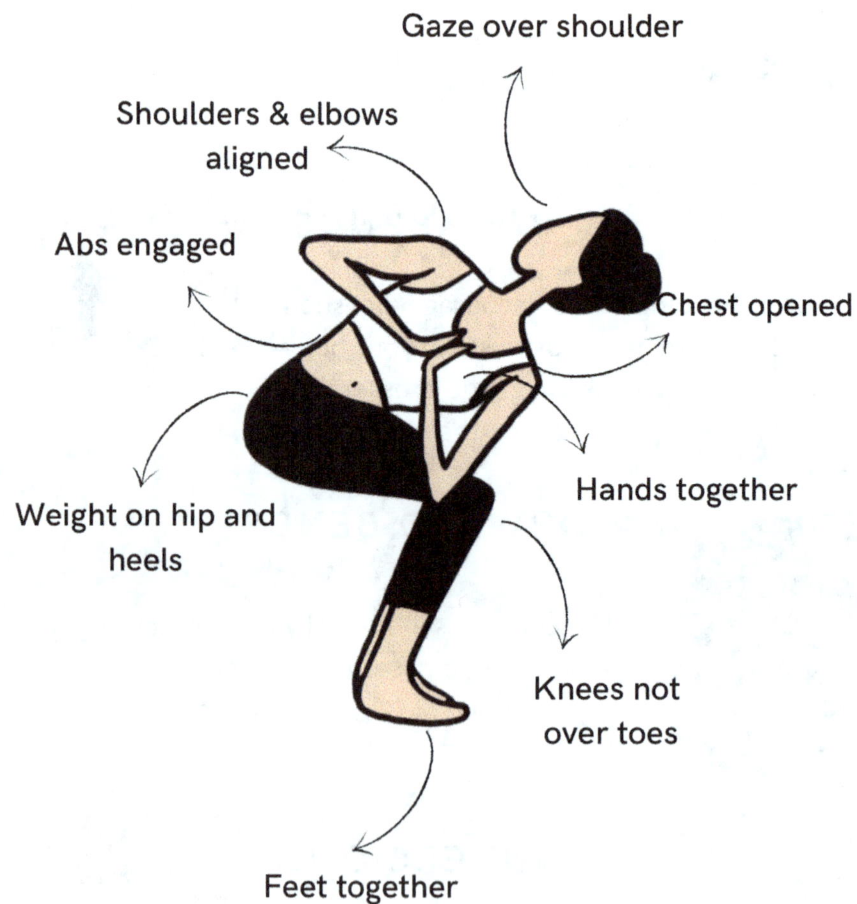

# Revolved Chair Pose

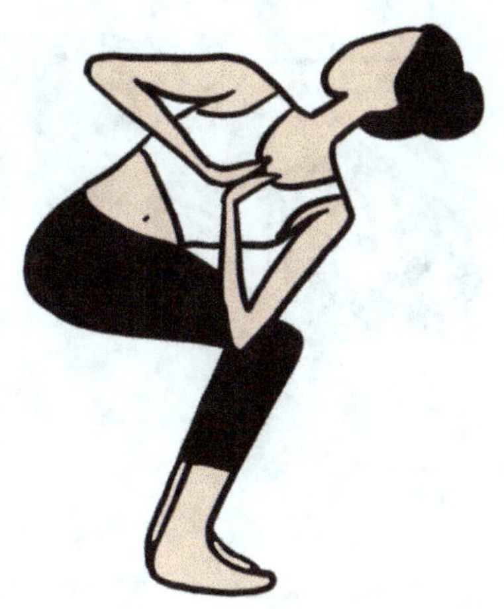

## How to:

1. Stand firm on the mat with your feet together.
2. Inhale, palms together in front of your chest (heart chakra) and engage your abs.
3. Exhale, bend your knees and make sure your knees are not over your toes.
4. Inhale, engage your abs.
5. Exhale, twist your upper body to your right, left elbow on your right thigh and your eyes gaze over the shoulder.

**Parivrtta Utkatasana**

# Revolved Chair Pose

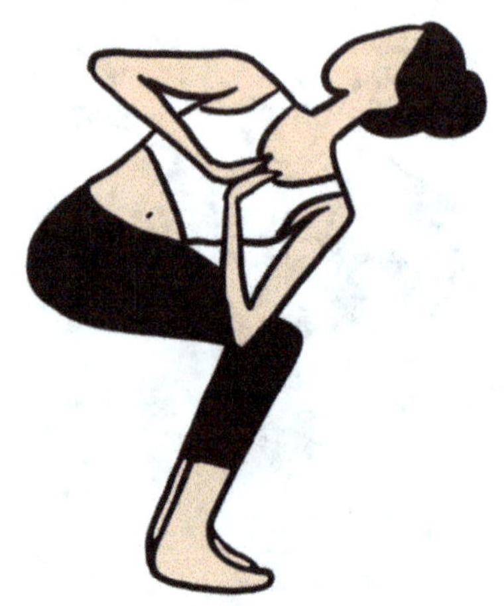

## Benefits

1. Opens chest, shoulders, and upper back.
2. Strengthens the hip flexor muscles, front and
   inner thighs.
1. Strengthens and stretches calf muscles.
2. Improves the sense of balance.
3. Stimulates abdominal organs and heart.

# Seated Twists Pose

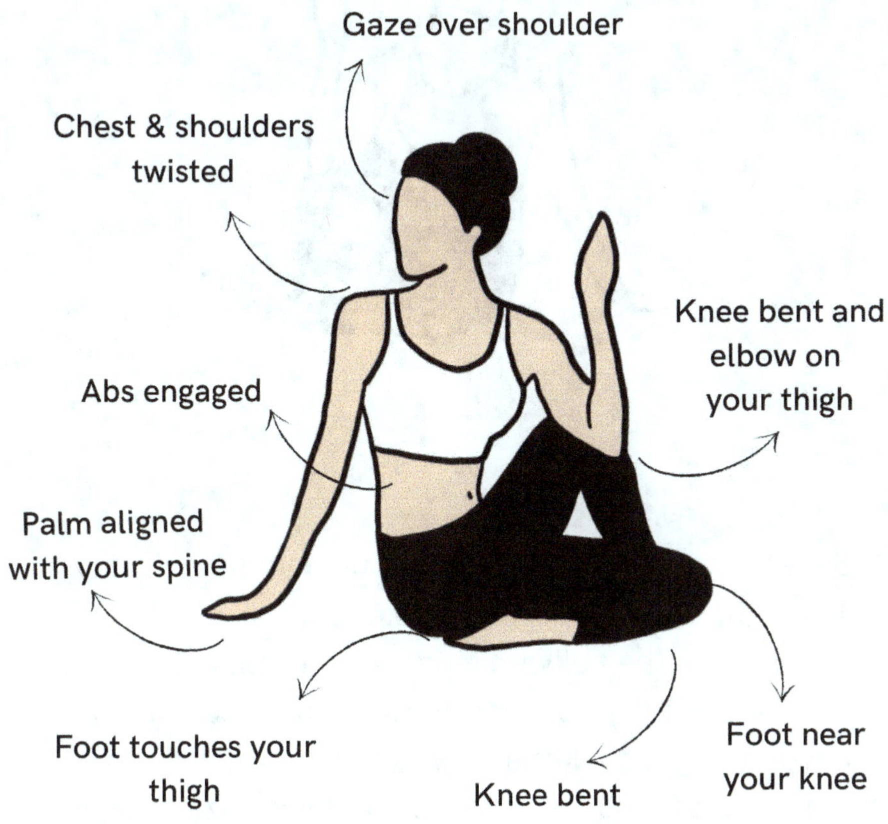

# Ardha Matsyendrasana
# Seated Twists Pose

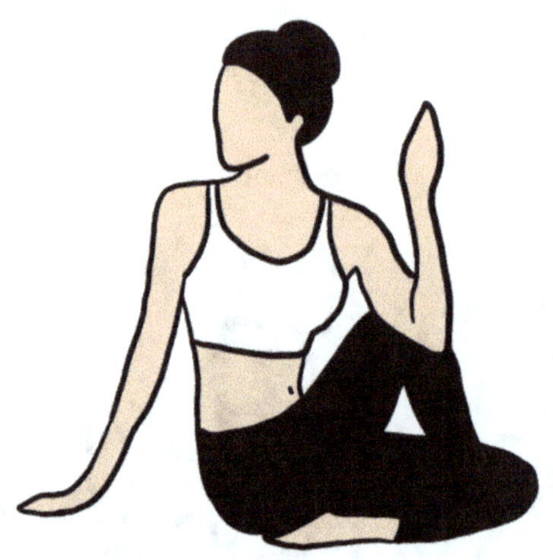

## How to:

1. Sit legs crossed. The left foot touching the right thigh. The right foot next to the left knee.
2. Inhale, tuck the belly in, lengthen the spine.
3. Exhale, twist the body to the right and place the right hand at the back, left elbow against the right thigh.
4. Inhale, chest and shoulders open, eyes gaze over the right shoulder.

# Seated Twists Pose

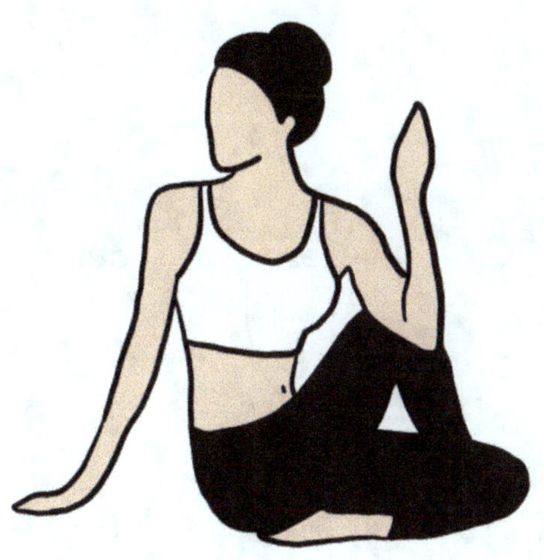

## Benefits

1. Releases the lower back muscles and provides relief from lower back pain.
2. Aids in maintaining normal rotation of your spinal cord.
3. Regulates your digestive system, thus improving digestion.
4. Helps relieve constipation.

# Spinal Twist Pose

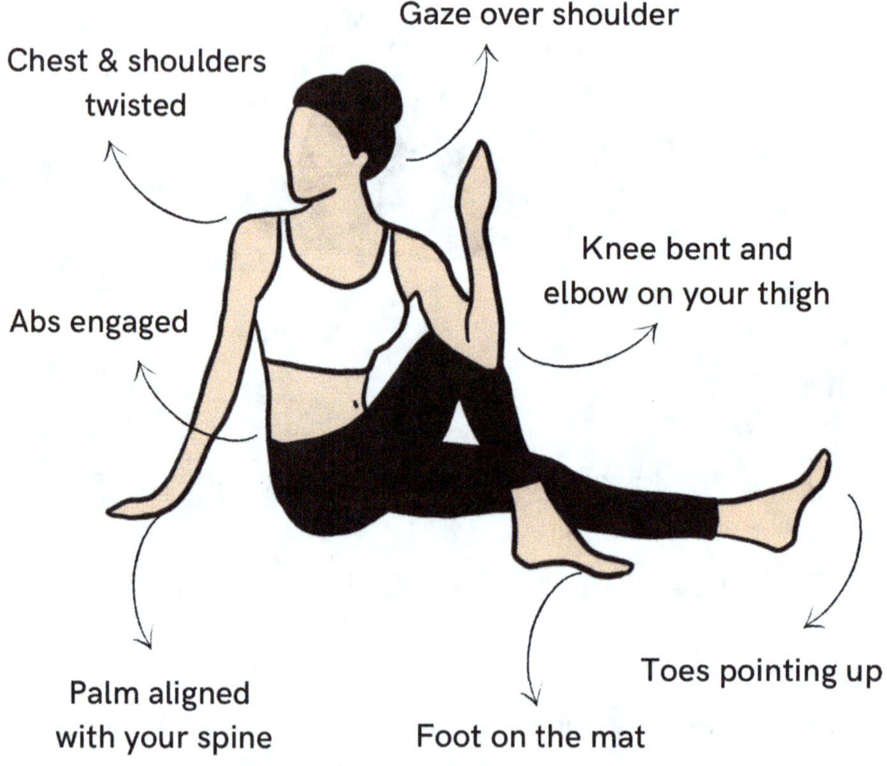

# Vakrasana
# Spinal Twist Pose

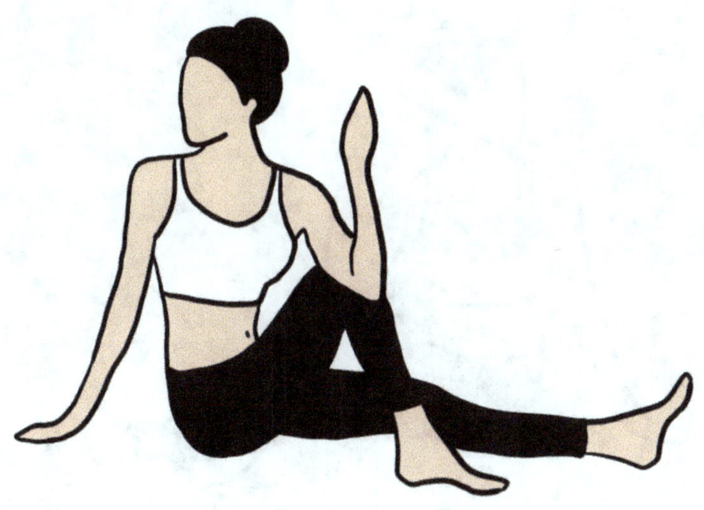

## How to:

1. Sit in Dandasana pose with your back straight. Bring your right knee up, right foot on the mat.
2. Inhale, tuck the belly in, lengthen the spine.
3. Exhale, twist the body to the right and place the right hand at the back, left elbow against the right thigh.
4. Inhale, chest and shoulders open, eyes gaze over the right shoulder.

# Spinal Twist Pose

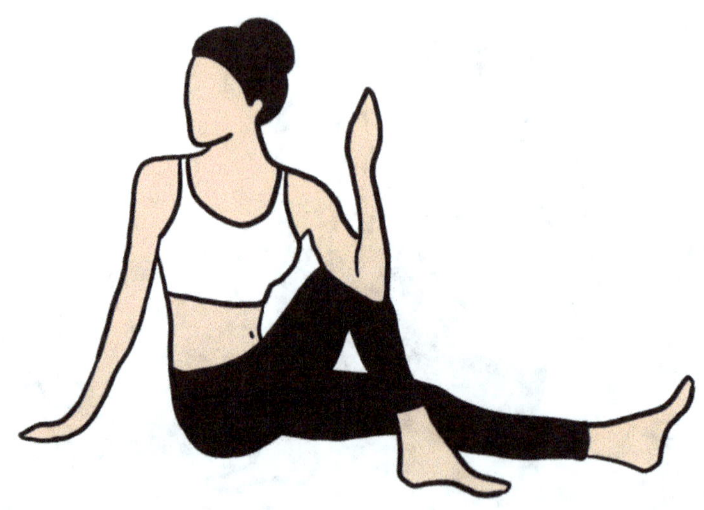

## Benefits

1. Helps relieve constipation and liver-related problems.
2. Releases the lower back muscles thereby providing relief from lower back pain.
3. Aids in maintaining normal rotation of your spinal cord.
4. Regulates your digestive system, thus improving digestion.

# Supine Spinal Twist Pose

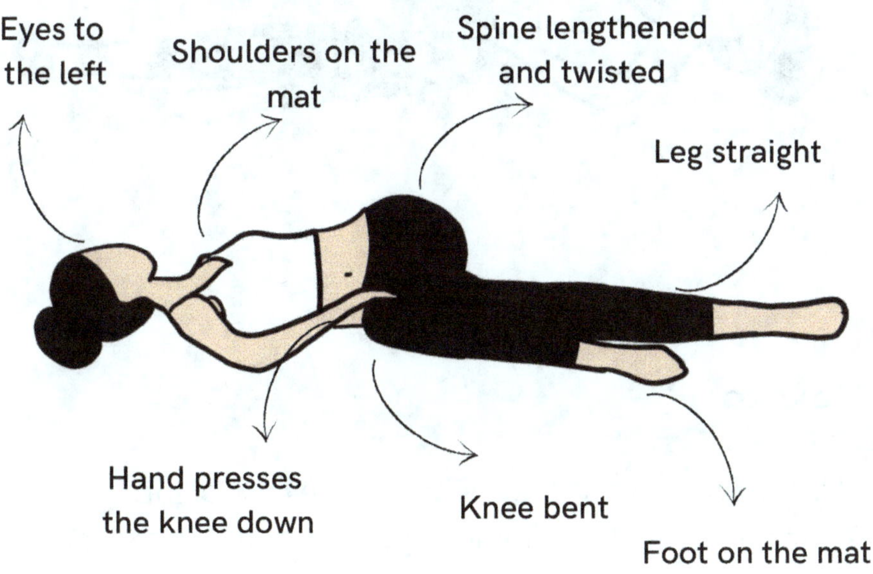

# Supine Spinal Twist Pose

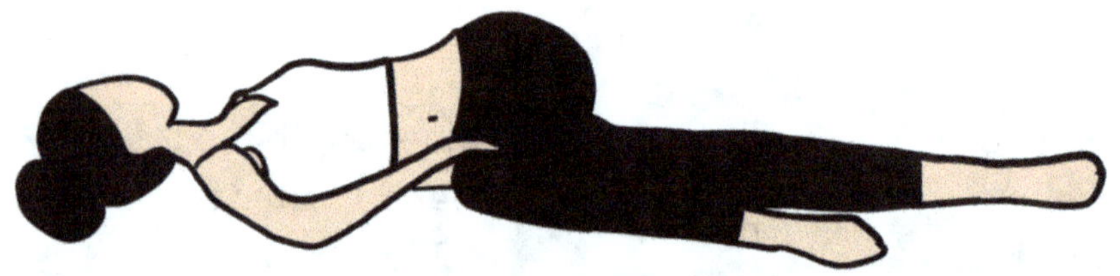

## How to:

1. Lie down on your back with both legs straight.
2. Inhale, bring the left knee up, right hand on the left knee.
3. Exhale, twist the body to the right. Left foot on the mat, knee turned to 90 degrees, look to the left and shoulders on the mat.

# Supine Spinal Twist Pose

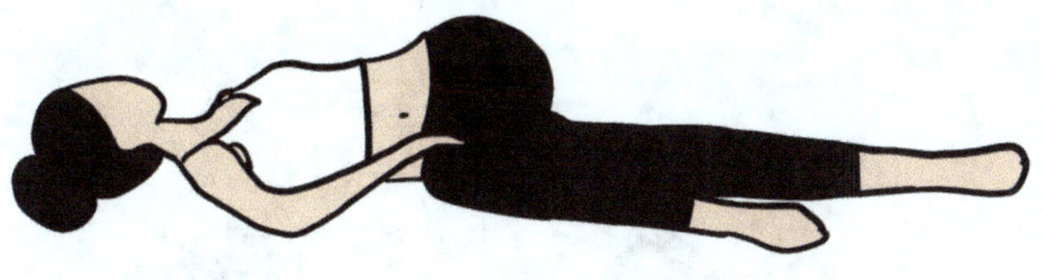

## Benefits

1. Helps release the lower back.
2. Improves spine mobility.
3. Opens tight shoulders.
4. Elongates the supporting spinal muscles.
5. Improves digestion and relieves constipation.
6. Quiets down the mind.

# Marjariasana
# Cat Pose

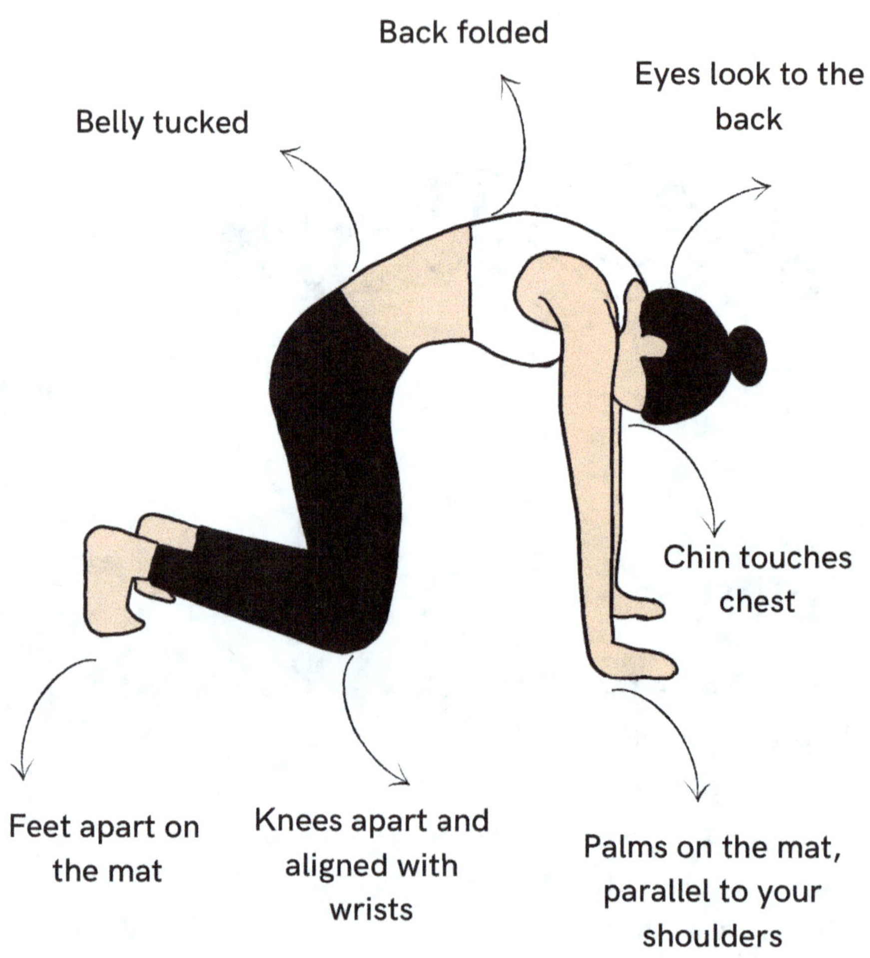

# Marjariasana
# Cat Pose

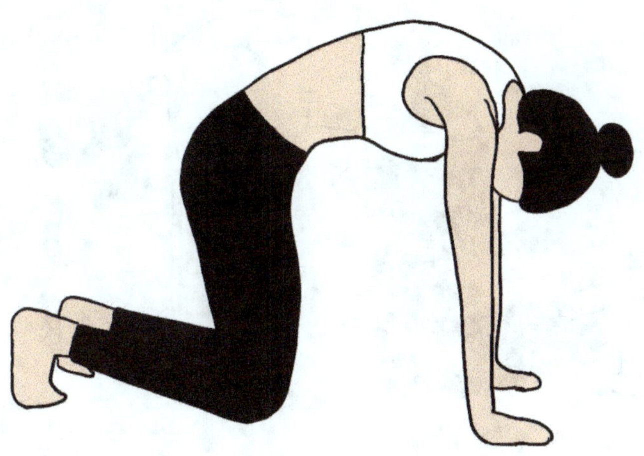

## How to:

1. Knees, palms and feet apart on the mat. Shoulders parallel with palms and knees aligned with the wrists.
2. Inhale, tuck the belly in, fold your back and your chin touches your chest. Eyes look to the back.

# Cat Pose

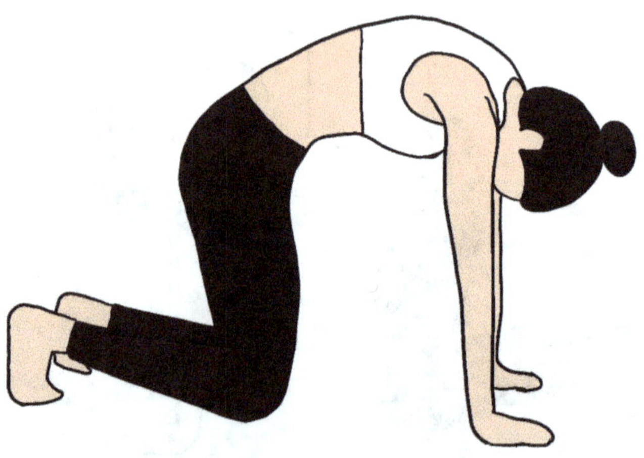

## Benefits

1. Helps relieve lower back pain.
2. Improve spine and hips mobility.
3. Enhances blood circulation as well as oxygen flow through the body.
4. Tones up the abs.
5. Improves digestion and relieves constipation.
6. Soothes menstrual cramps in women.

# Bitilasana
# Cow Pose

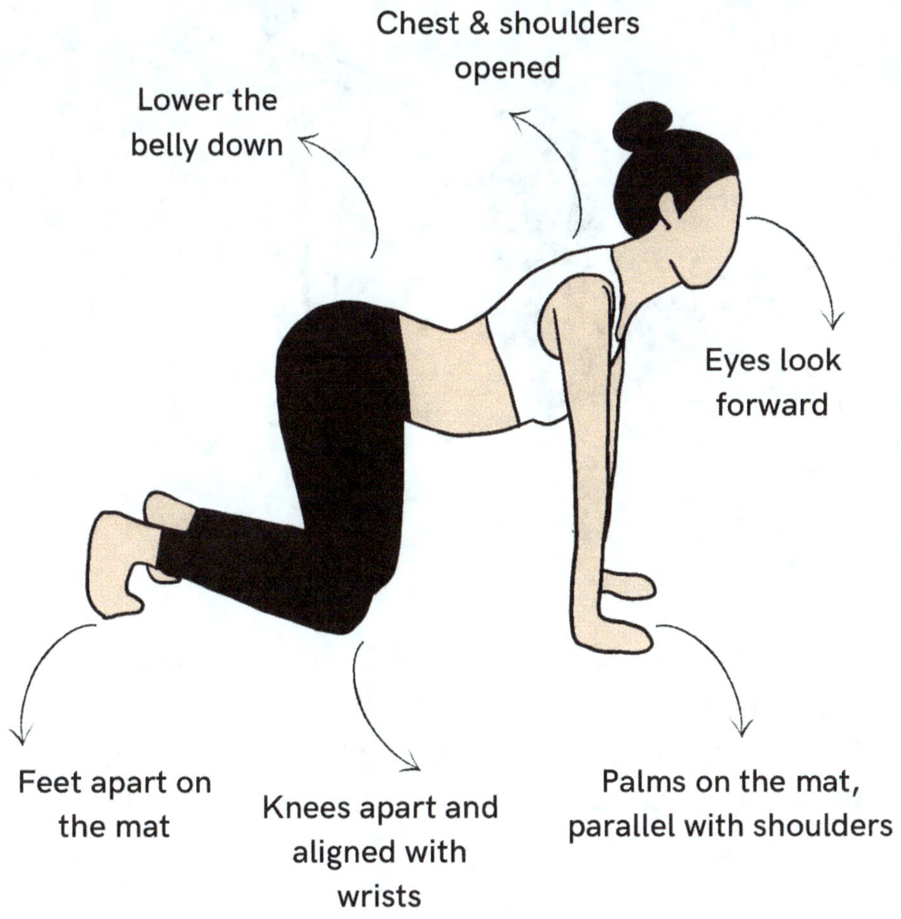

# Cow Pose

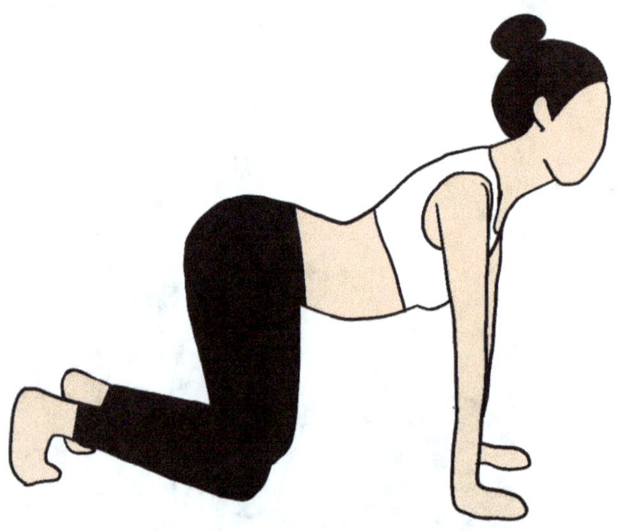

## How to:

1. Knees, palms and feet apart on the mat. Shoulders parallel with palms and knees aligned with the wrists.
2. Inhale, then exhale and lower the belly down, lengthen the torso. Shoulders and chest opened, eyes look forward.

# Bitilasana
# Cow Pose

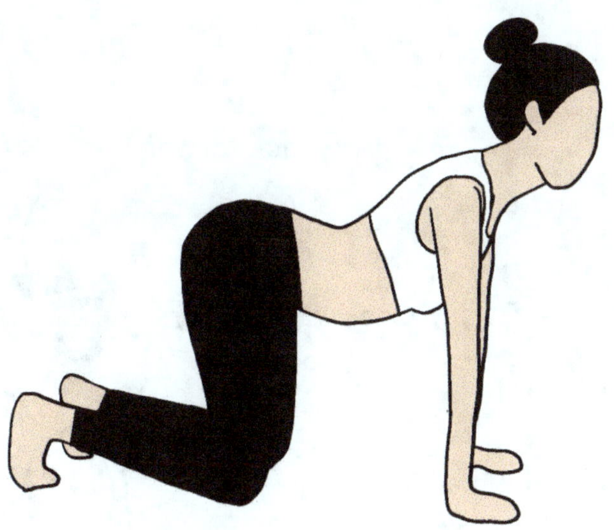

## Benefits

1. Helps release tension at lower back and improve spine and hips mobility.
2. Relieves tensions around the lower back, middle back, neck and shoulders.
3. Improves digestion and relieves constipation.
4. Soothes menstrual cramps in women.

# Cobra Pose

Eyes look forward
Chest & shoulders opened
Legs on the mat
Feet together
Palms firmly on the mat with fingers apart
Belly & torso lengthened

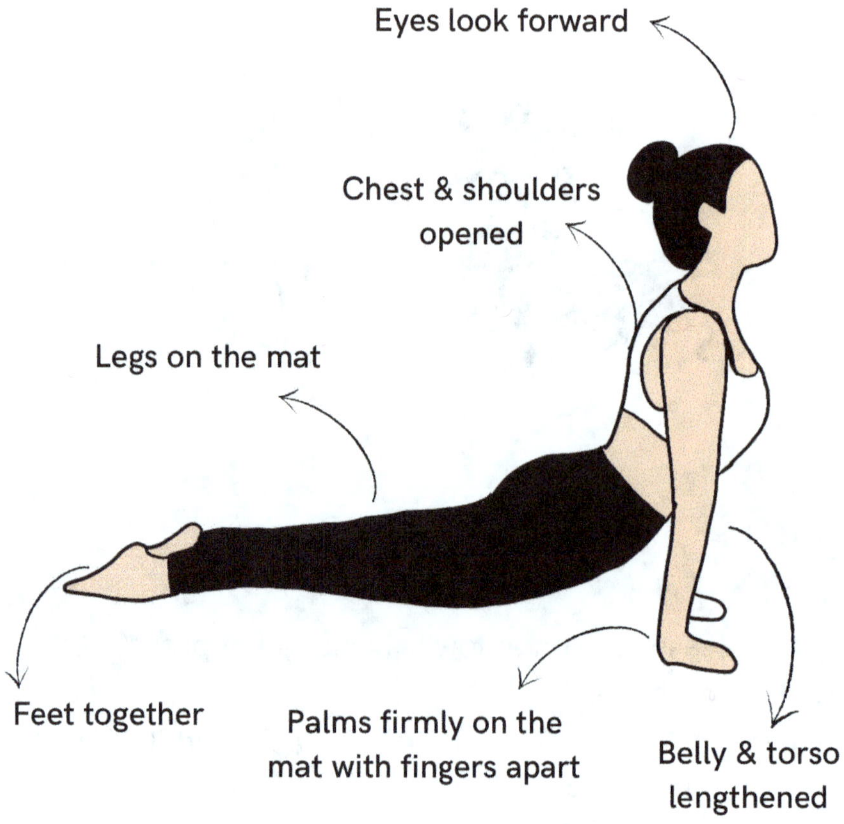

# Cobra Pose

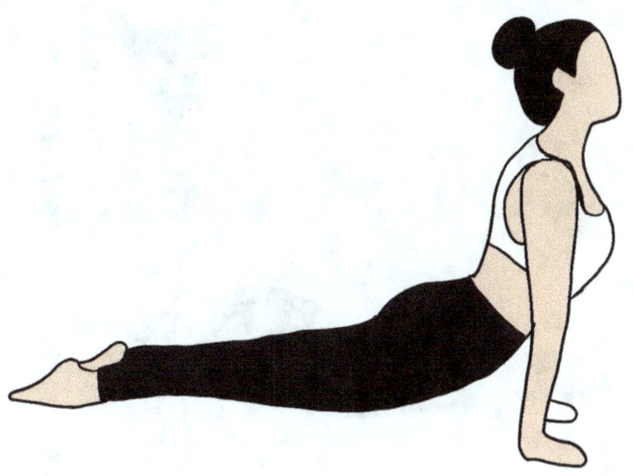

## How to:

1. Lie down on your front with your feet together. Place your palms firmly on the mat with fingers apart next to your chest.
2. Inhale, press your palms firmly on the mat and slide your body up.
3. Exhale, roll your shoulders open, lengthen your torso and your eyes look forward or look up.

# Bhujangasana
# Cobra Pose

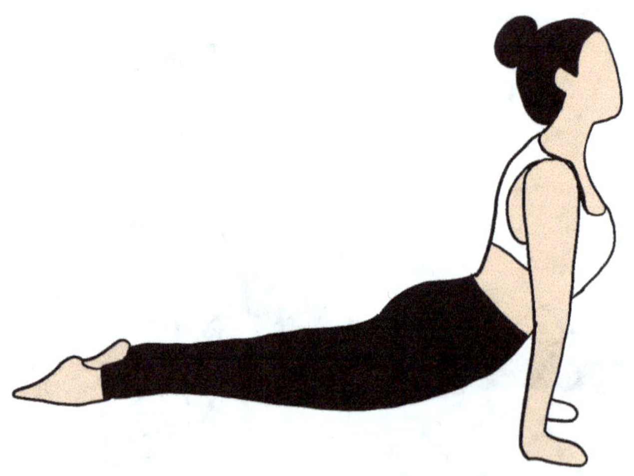

## Benefits

1. Strengthens the spine and tones the buttocks.
2. Stimulates abdominal organs and cures constipation.
3. Soothes sciatica.
4. Therapeutic for asthma.

# Ardha Ustrasana
# Half Camel Pose

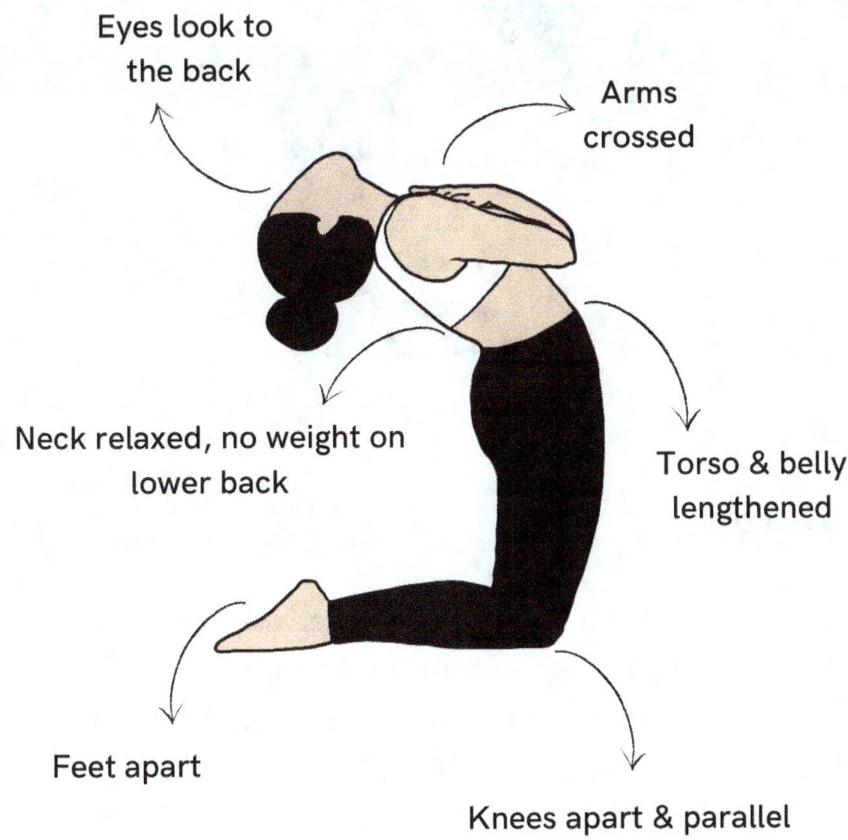

# Half Camel Pose

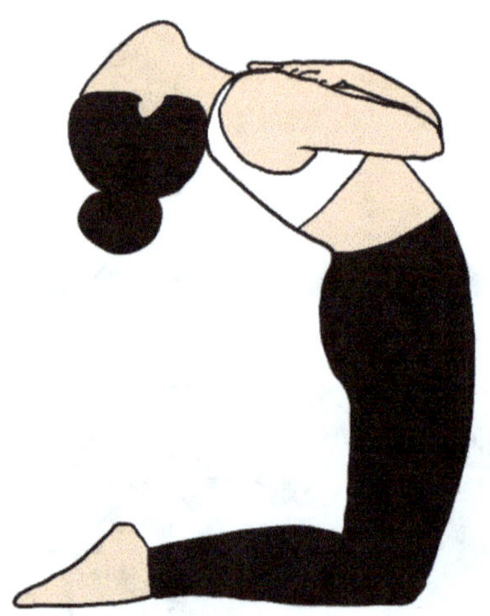

## How to:

1. Stand on your knees with your knees being parallel with your hips. Toes or feet on the mat.
2. Inhale, palms crossed, hands on shoulders. Tuck your belly in and engage your buttocks.
3. Exhale, lengthen your torso and your neck. Your eyes look to the back.

## Ardha Ustrasana
# Half Camel Pose

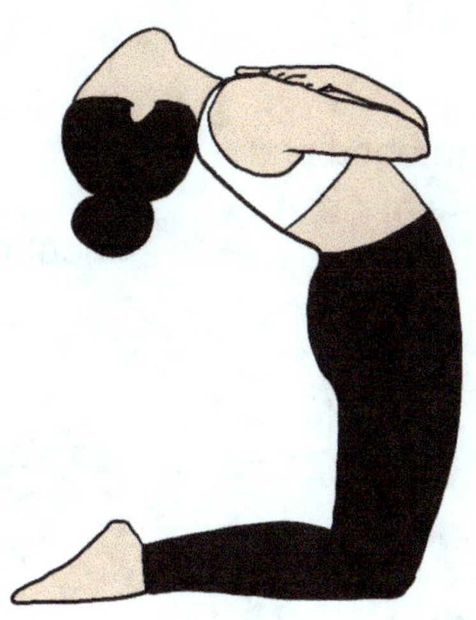

## Benefits

1. Opens the chest and upper body.
2. Stimulates the digestive and respiratory systems.
3. Strengthens and stretches the back muscles.
4. Stimulates the thyroid gland.
5. Aids digestion while toning core muscles.

# Ardha Uttanasana
# Half Forward Bend Pose

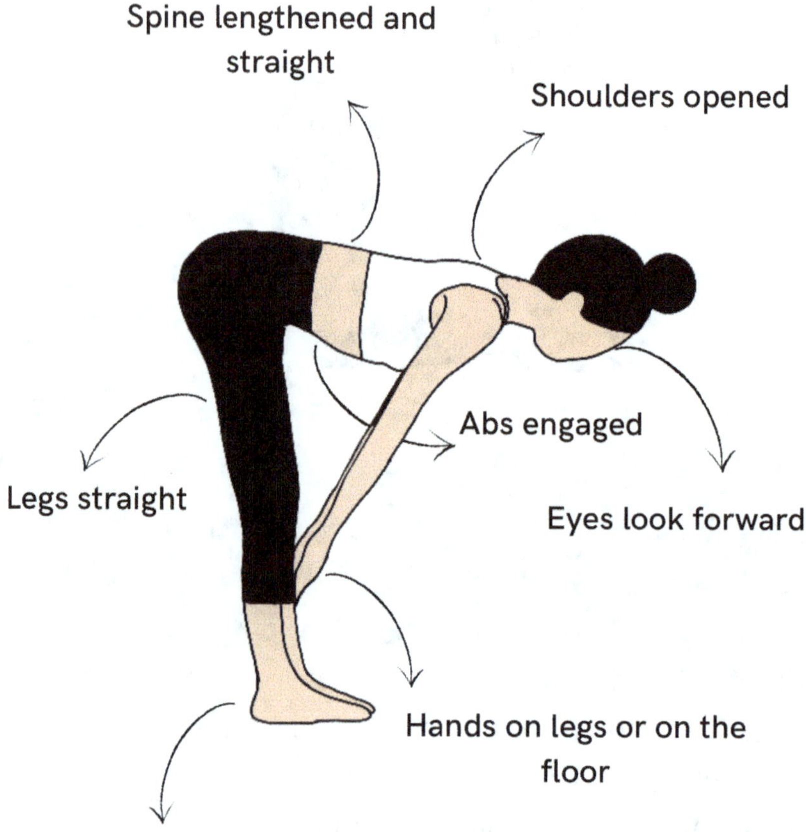

# Ardha Uttanasana
# Half Forward Bend Pose

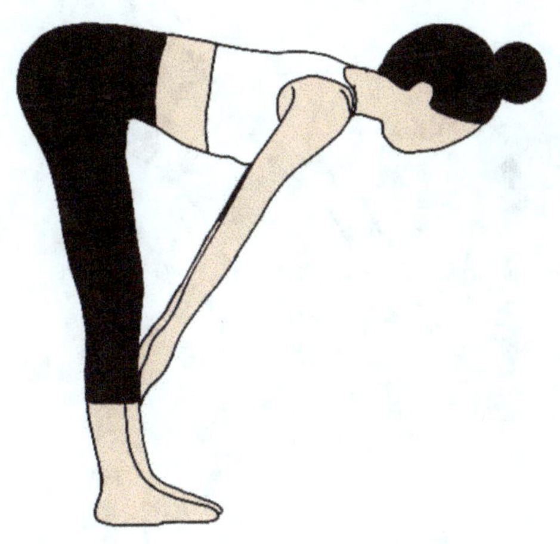

## How to:

1. Stand tall on the mat with your feet together.
2. Engage your legs, abs and buttocks.
3. Lengthen your spine and roll your shoulders open.
4. Inhale, raise your palms up in the air.
5. Exhale, bend forward and place your palms on your legs or on the mat.
6. Inhale, roll your shoulders open.
7. Exhale, your eyes look forward.

# Half Forward Bend Pose

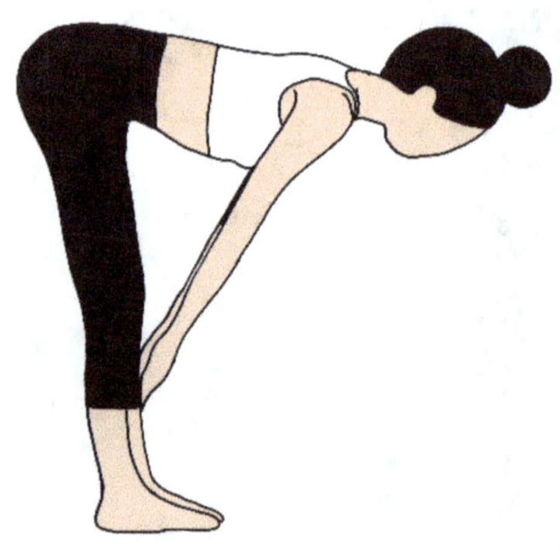

## Benefits

1. Stretches the torso, spine, hamstrings, and calves.
2. Strengthens the back and improves posture.
3. Stimulates the digestive organs.

# Pyramid Pose

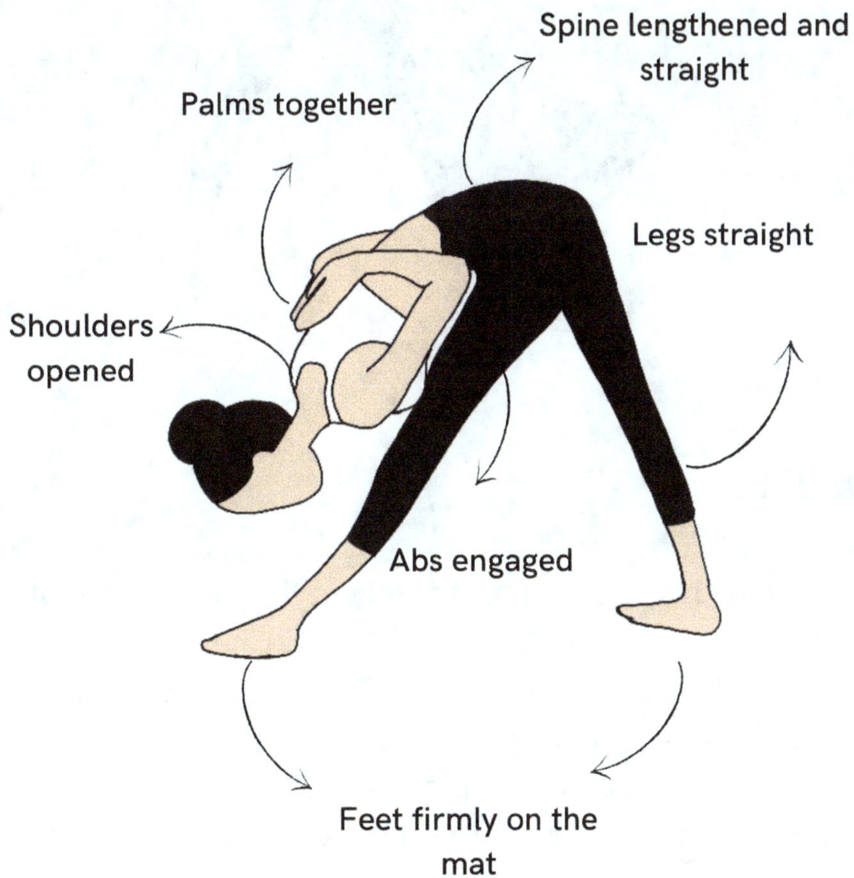

# Parsvottanasana
# Pyramid Pose

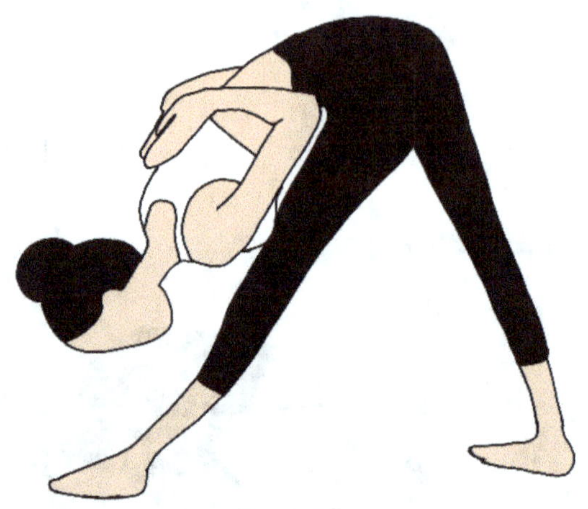

## How to:

1. Begin by placing your feet firmly at the top of the mat.
2. Step your right foot back 2 to 4 feet. Line up heel to heel with your back foot at a 30- to 45-degree angle.
3. Inhale, spread your arms out to the sides. Exhale, bring your palms together behind your back. If this is too difficult, place your palms on the block or your palms touch in front of your chest.

# Parsvottanasana
# Pyramid Pose

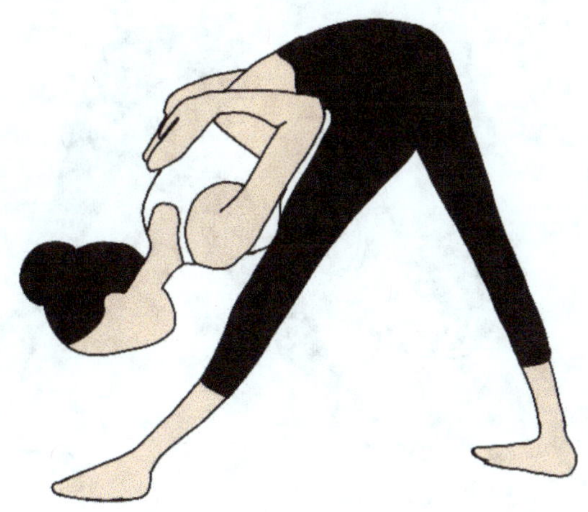

## How to:

4. Inhale, lengthen your spine, tuck your belly in and engage your quadriceps.
5. Exhale, slowly bend forward, your chest touching your thigh, chin touching your knee and your eyes look forward.

# Pyramid Pose

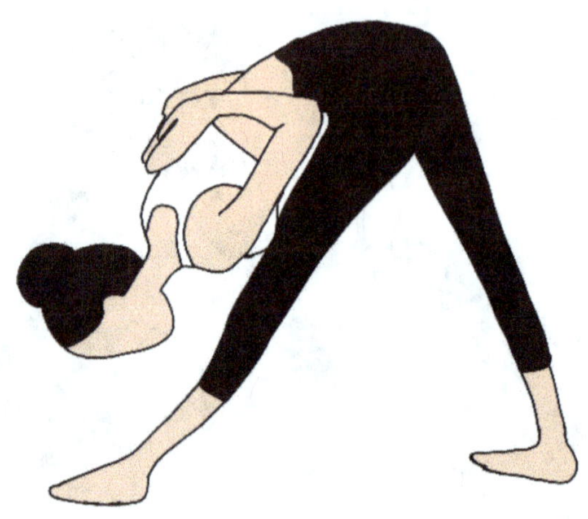

## Benefits

1. Stretches hamstrings and lengthens your spine.
2. Strengthens quads, calves, ankles and feet.
3. Opens chest and shoulders.
4. Stimulates the digestive system.

# Prasarita Padottanasana
# Wide Legged Standing Forward Bend Pose

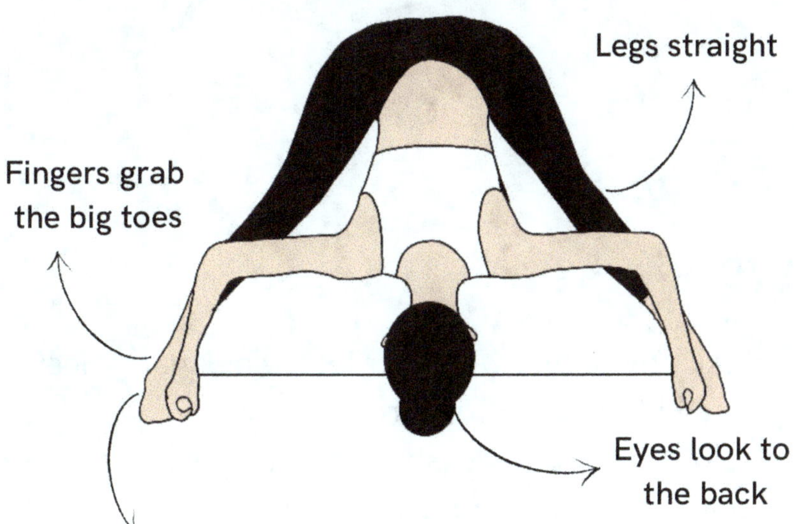

# Wide Legged Standing Forward Bend Pose

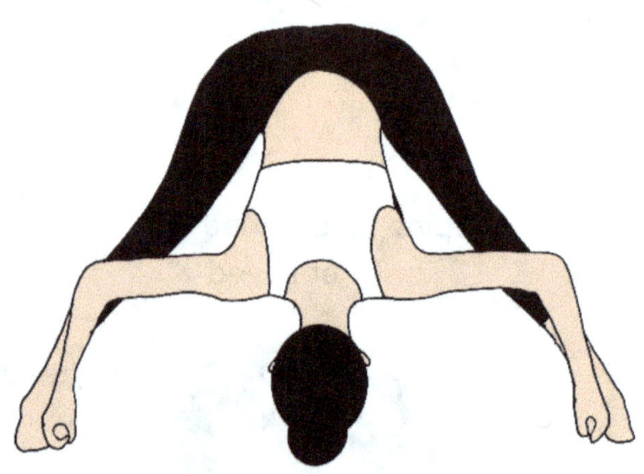

## How to:

1. Stand tall on the mat with your legs wide apart. Heels aligned and toes point forward.
2. Inhale, engage your legs, abs and buttocks. Lengthen your spine and roll your shoulders open.
3. Exhale, bend forward, your fingers hook the big toes or place your palms on the mat.

# Wide Legged Standing Forward Bend Pose

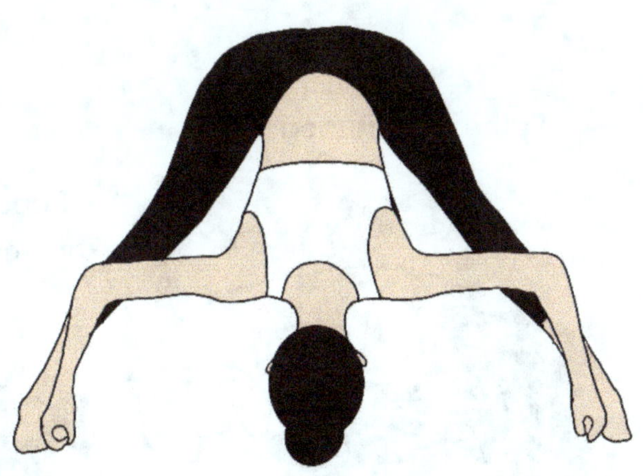

## Benefits

1. Stretches lower back, hamstrings and calves.
2. Strengthens the back and improves posture.
3. Stimulates the digestive organs.
4. Improves circulation.
5. Reduces stress and anxiety.

# Balasana
# Child's Pose

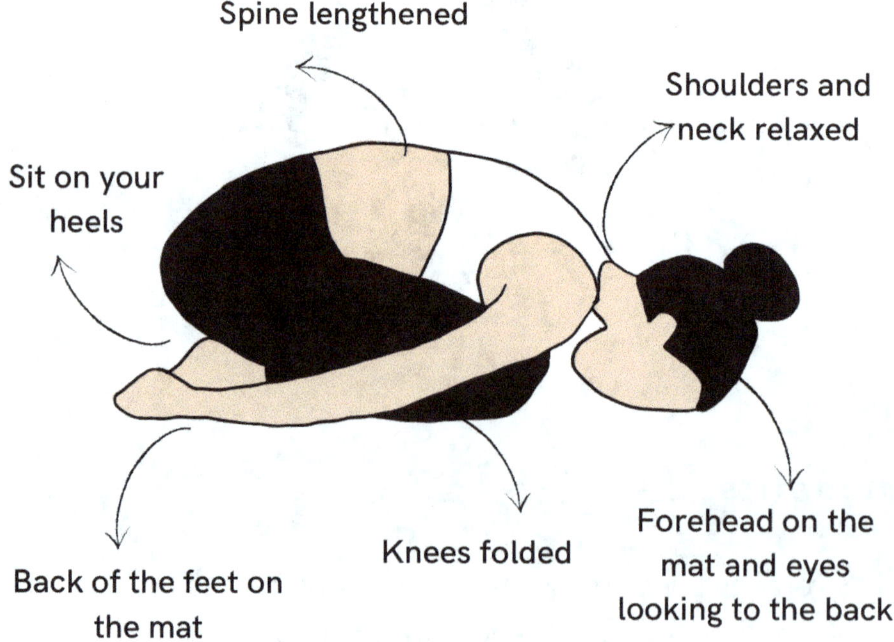

# Balasana
# Child's Pose

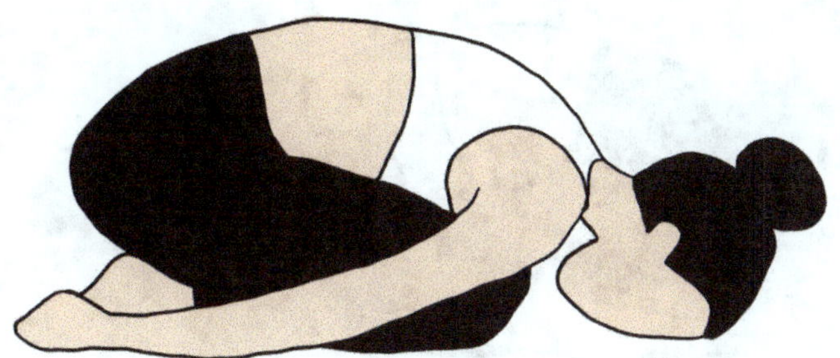

## How to:

1. Sit down on your heels with your feet on the mat.
   Keep your knees together or apart.
1. Inhale, your back straight and your abs engaged.
2. Exhale, slowly bend forward, place your forehead on
   the mat. Stretch your arms forward or toward the back.

# Balasana
# Child's Pose

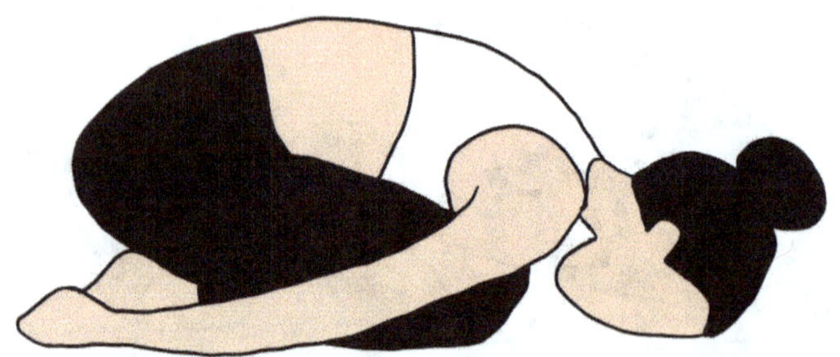

## Benefits

1. Stretches back, hips, thighs and ankles
2. Relieves back pain.
3. Stimulates the digestive organs.
4. Normalises circulation.

# Adho Mukha Svanasana
# Downward Dog Pose

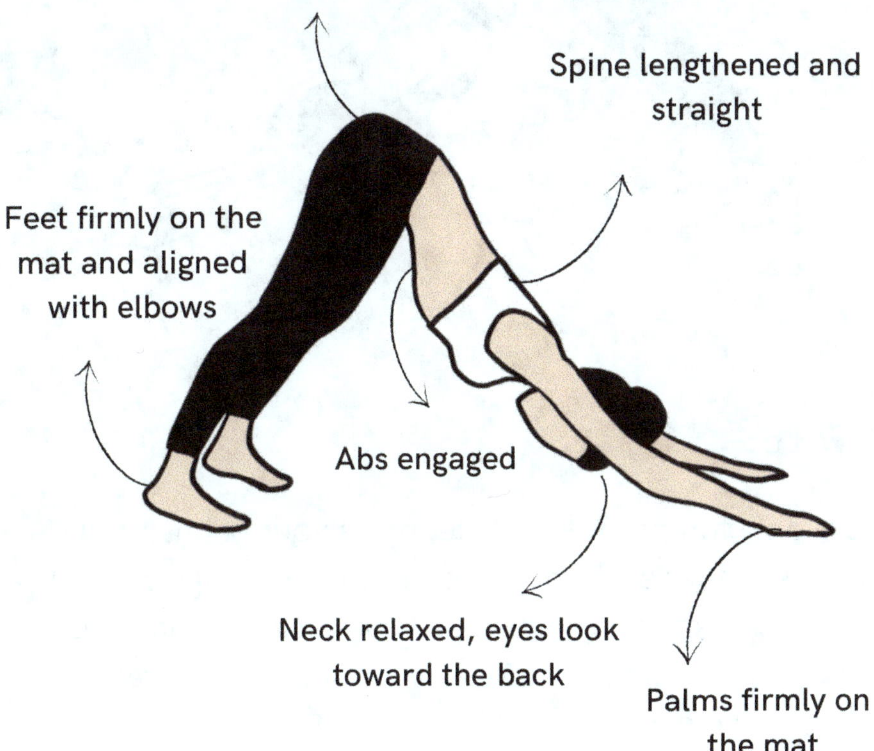

# Adho Mukha Svanasana
# Downward Dog Pose

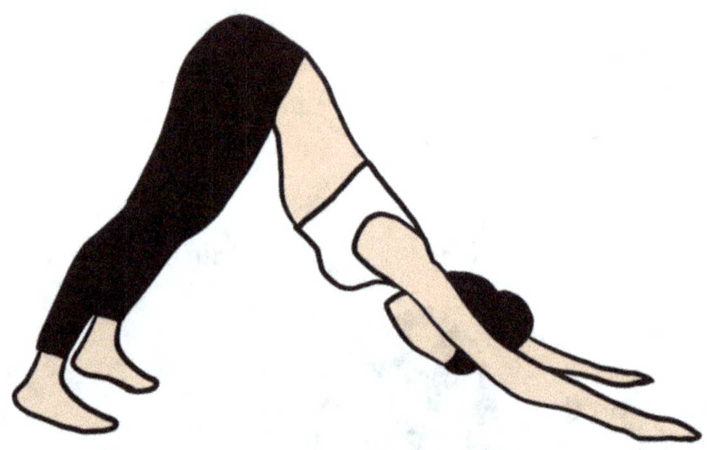

## How to:

1. On table top position, inhale, press your palms firmly on the mat and lift your hips up with your legs straight.
2. Exhale, push your hips toward the back and place your feet firmly on the mat. Relax your neck, your eyes look toward the back.
3. Engage your core and hold the pose for 3-5 breaths.

# Downward Dog Pose

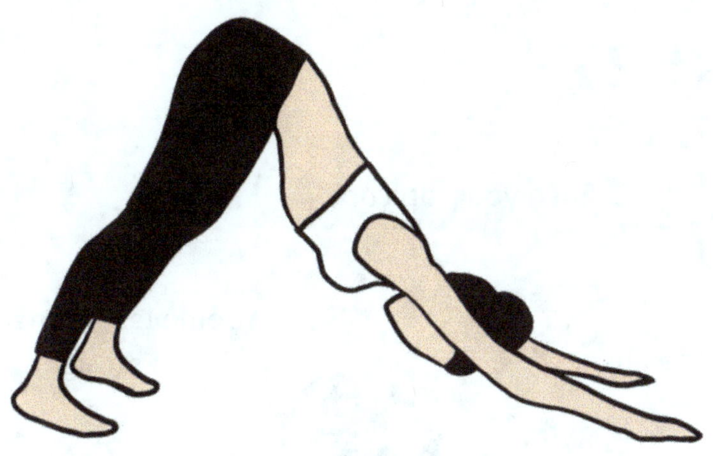

## Benefits

1. Calms the brain and helps relieve stress and mild depression.
2. Stretches the shoulders, hamstrings, calves, and arches.
3. Strengthens the arms, shoulders and legs.
4. Improves blood circulation.
5. Improves digestion.
6. Alleviates pain in the lower back.

# Ardha Pincha Mayurasana
## Dolphin Pose

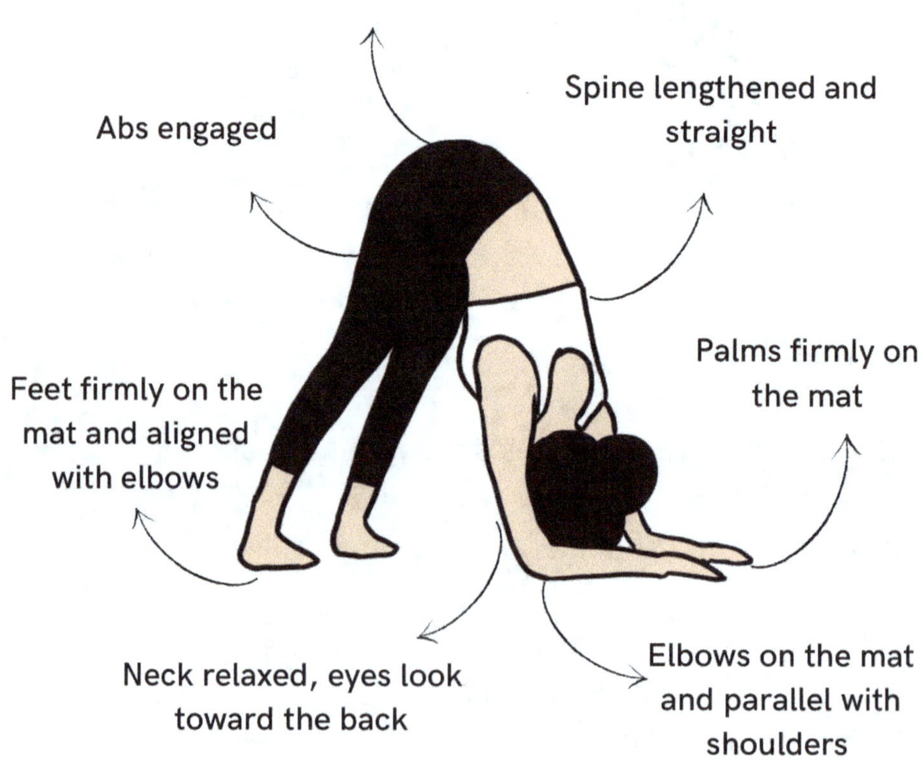

# Dolphin Pose

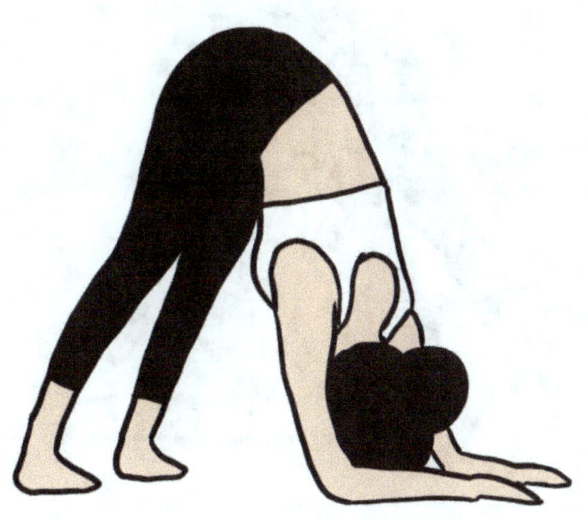

## How to:

1. On table top position, place your forearms on the mat.
2. Inhale, lift your hips up with your legs straight.
3. Exhale, push your hips toward the back and place your feet firmly on the mat. Relax your neck and eyes look toward the back.
4. Engage your core and hold the pose for 3-5 breaths.

# Dolphin Pose

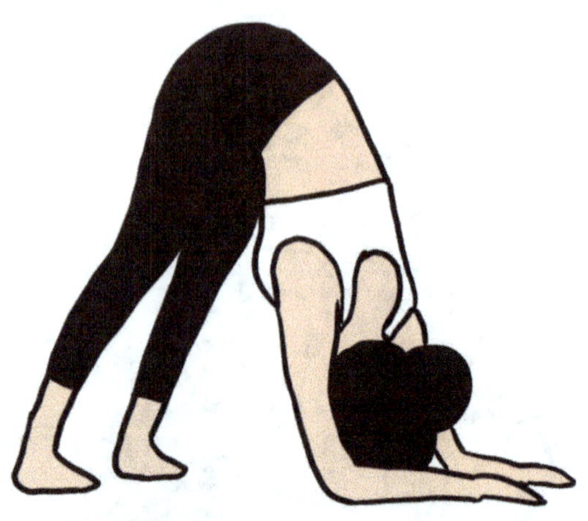

## Benefits

1. Calms the brain and helps relieve stress and mild depression.
2. Stretches the shoulders, hamstrings, calves, and arches.
3. Strengthens the arms and legs.
4. Helps relieve the symptoms of menopause.
5. Improves digestion.
6. Relieves headache, insomnia, back pain, and fatigue.
7. Therapeutic for high blood pressure, asthma, flat feet, and sciatica.

# Shoulders Stand Pose

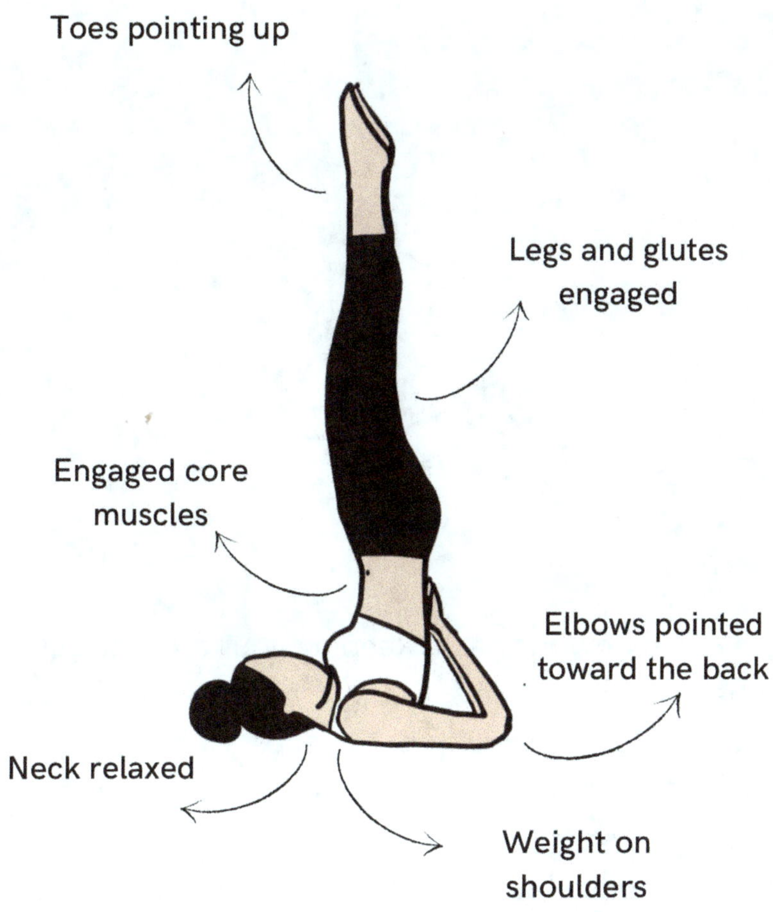

# Shoulders Stand Pose

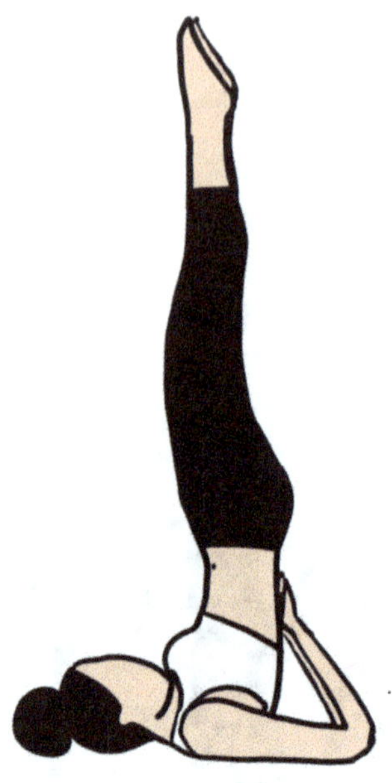

## How to:

1. Lie down on your back, keeping your arms straight.
2. Inhale, engage your core then raise your legs up and support your back with both hands.
3. Exhale, relax your neck and shoulders, pointing your toes up to the sky.
4. Hold the pose for 3-5 breaths with your core and legs engaged.

# Shoulders Stand Pose

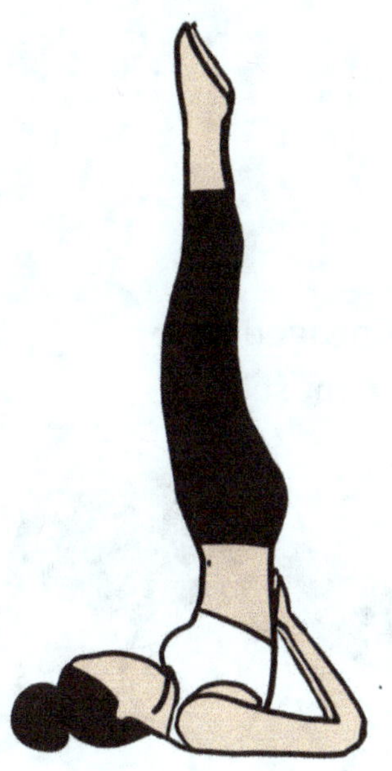

## Benefits

1. Stretches shoulders and neck.
2. Increases circulation towards the neck, face, head and brain.
3. Stimulates bowel movements and clears up digestive system.
4. Enhances lymphatic system.
5. Relieves stress and anxiety.
6. Cures Epilepsy and sperm disorders.

# Halasana
# Plow Pose

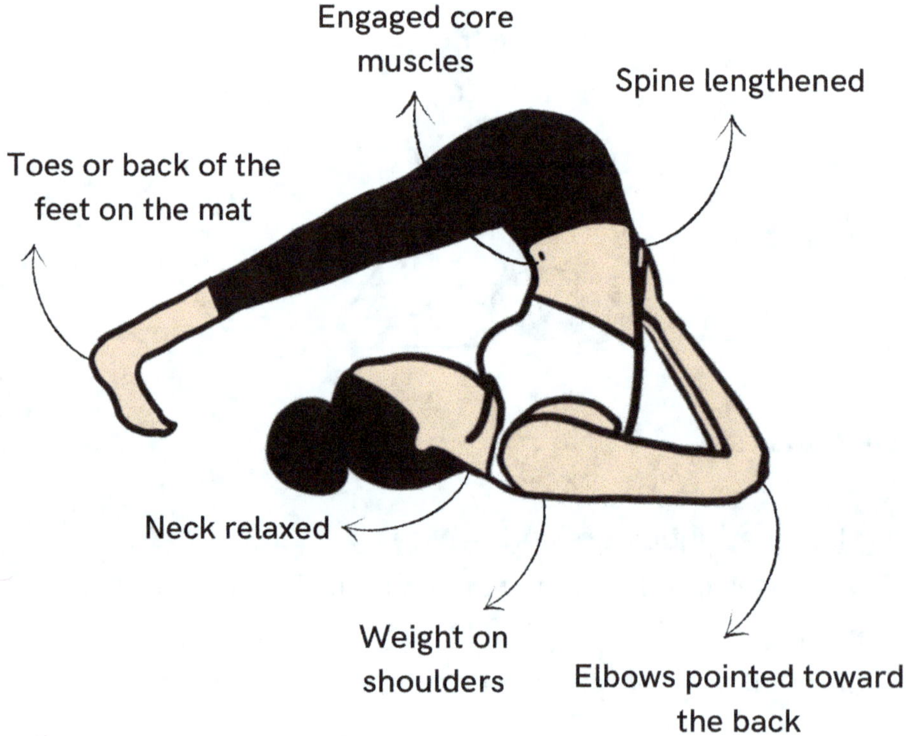

# Plow Pose

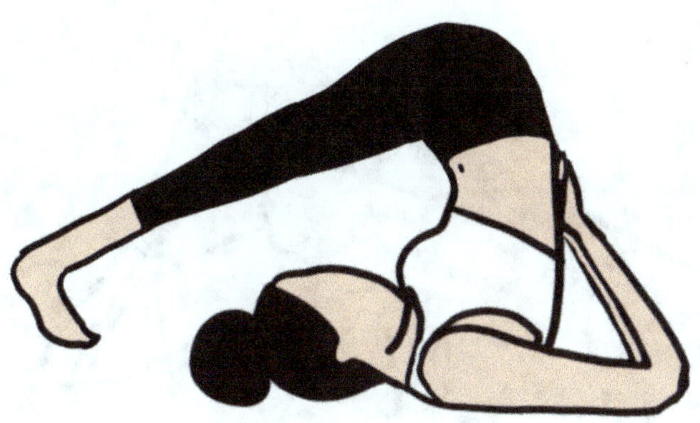

## How to:

1. Lie down on your back, keeping your arms straight.
2. Inhale, engage your core then raise your legs up and support your back with both hands.
3. Exhale, drop your legs toward the back, place your toes or the back of your feet on the mat.
4. Inhale, lengthen your spine and stretch and engage your legs.
5. Exhale, relax your neck and shoulders. Hold the pose for 3-5 breaths.

# Halasana
# Plow Pose

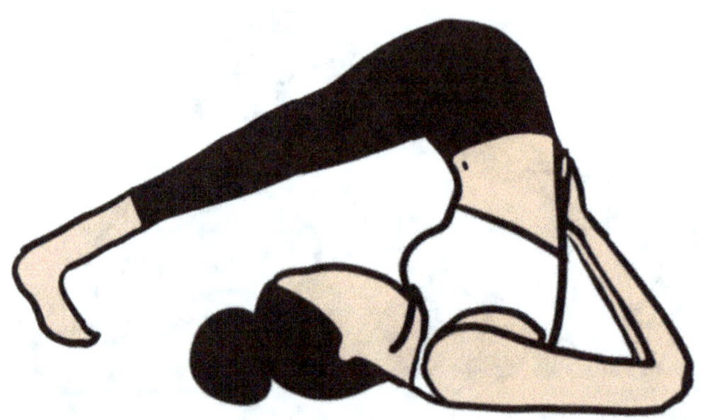

## Benefits

1. Strengthens and opens up the neck, shoulders, abs and back muscles.
2. Calms the nervous system, reduces stress and fatigue.
3. Tones the legs and improves leg flexibility.
4. Stimulates bowel movements and clears up digestive system.
5. Stimulates the thyroid gland and strengthens the immune system.

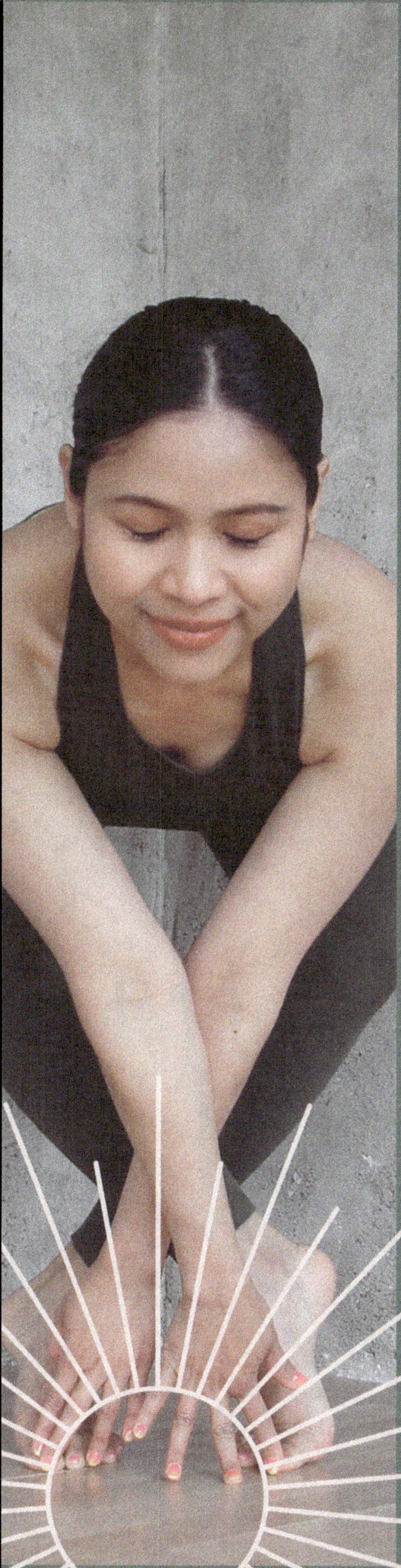

# DETOX YOGA FLOW

Learn how to flow effortlessly to detox your body with different yoga poses which help improve the detoxifying organs.

# DETOX FLOW A
## 8 YOGA POSES

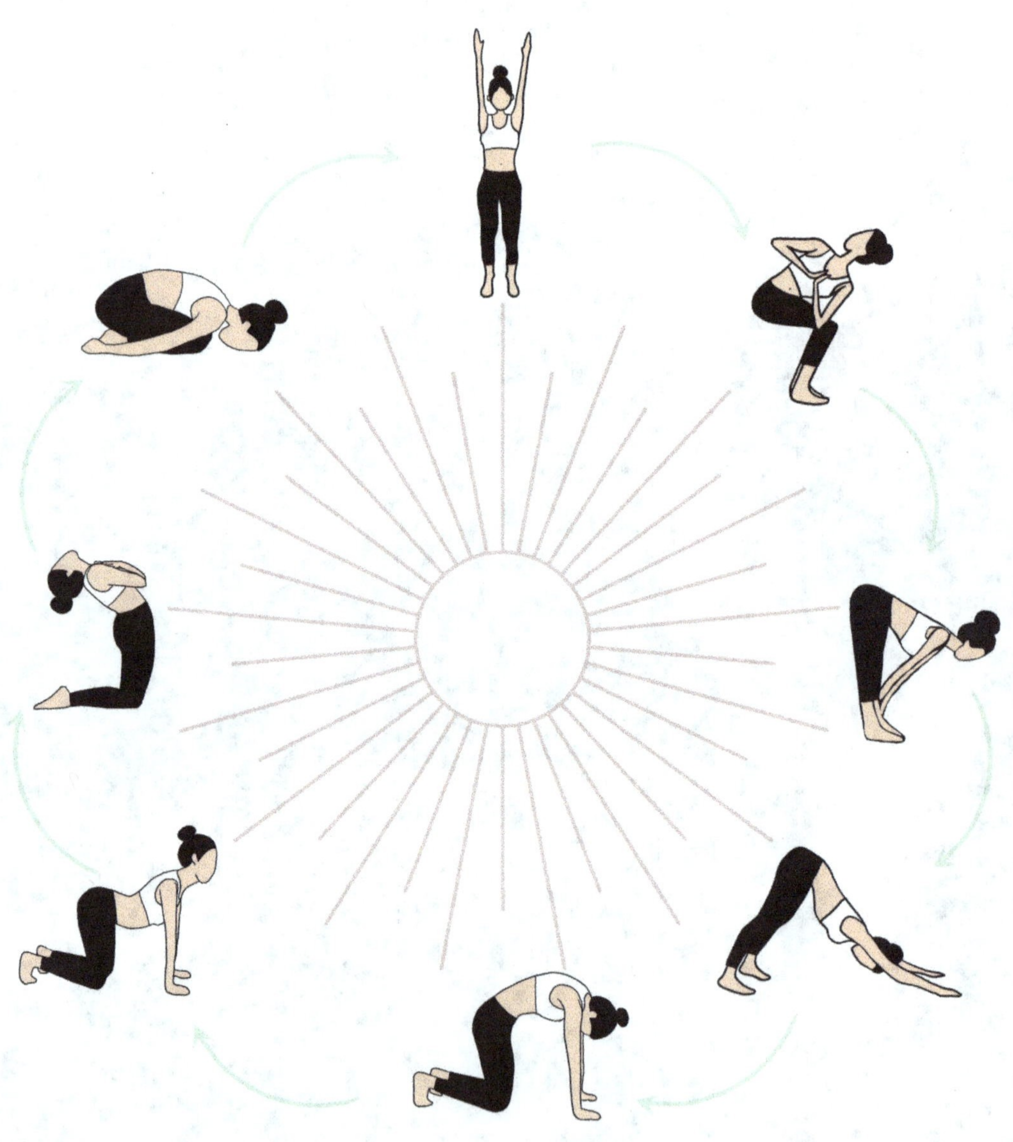

# DETOX FLOW A
## 8 YOGA POSES

**Step 1:**

Stand tall, feet apart with your legs, glutes and abs engaged.

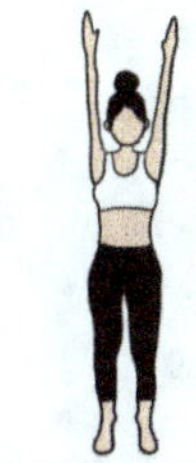

★ **Step 2 :**

Inhale, raise your palms and your heels up.

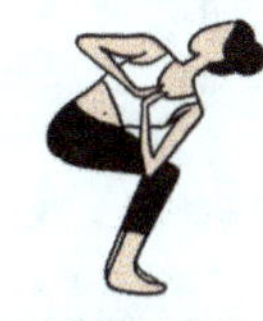

★ **Step 3 :**

Exhale, heels on the mat and bend your knees. Palms together at your chest and twist your spine to the right.

**Step 6 :**

Inhale, return your body to the centre and your legs straight.

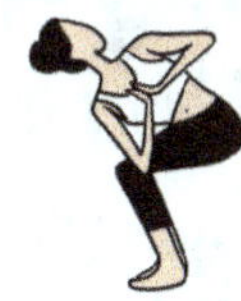

★ **Step 5 :**

Exhale, twist your body to the left.

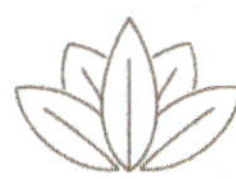

**Step 4 :**

Inhale, return your body to the centre.

★ Hold the pose for 5-10 breaths

# DETOX FLOW A
## 8 YOGA POSES

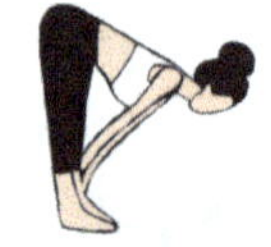

⭐ **Step 7:**

Exhale, bend forward, your fingers touch the mat or your palms on your legs.

**Step 8 :**

Inhale, press your palms on the mat firmly, then step your legs to the back or jump to the back.

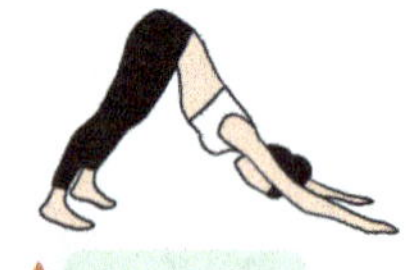

⭐ **Step 9 :**

Exhale, your feet on the mat, then push your hips toward the back.

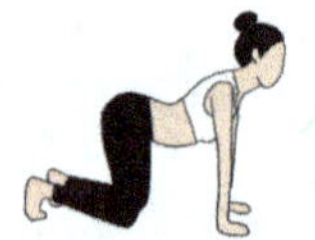

⭐ **Step 12 :**

Exhale, lower your belly down, lengthen your chest and your eyes look forward.

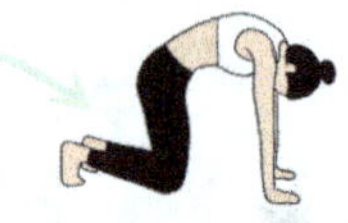

⭐ **Step 11 :**

Inhale, tuck your belly in, round your back, your chin touching your chest.

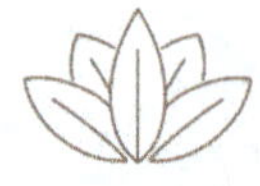

**Step 10 :**

Inhale, your eyes look forward. Exhale, place your knees down on the mat.

You can repeat this sequence 2-3 rounds.

⭐ Hold the pose for 5-10 breaths

# DETOX FLOW A
## 8 YOGA POSES

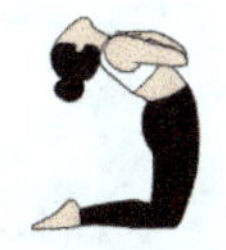

★ Step 13:

Inhale, stand on your knees and lengthen your chest toward the back. Exhale, push your hips forward.

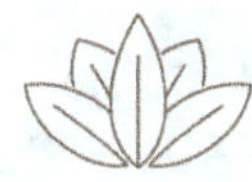

Step 14 :

Inhale, bring your body back to the centre.

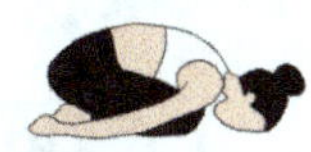

★ Step 15 :

Exhale, sit on your heels and bend forward. Your forehead is on the mat.

## ...DO THIS IF YOU WANT TO FLOW MORE...

Add the following poses after step 13, then repeat the flow as many times as you like. Resume step 14 - 15 when you want to end the flow or continue to Flow B.

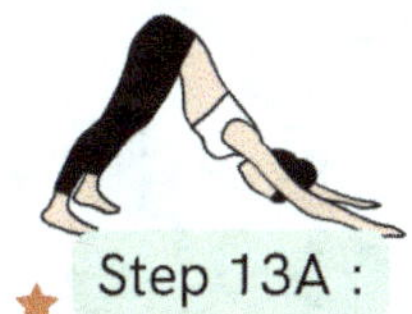

★ Step 13A :

Exhale, place your palms on the mat firmly. Inhale, lift your hips up. Exhale, push your hips toward the back.

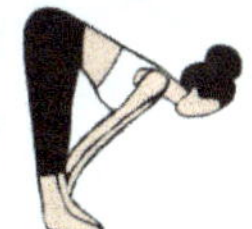

★ Step 13B :

Inhale, step forward or jump forward. Exhale, legs straight.

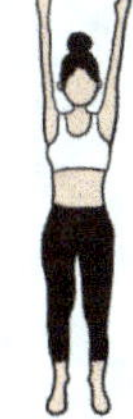

★ Step 13C :

Inhale, raise your palms and your heels up.

★ Hold the pose for 5-10 breaths

# DETOX FLOW B
## 8 YOGA POSES

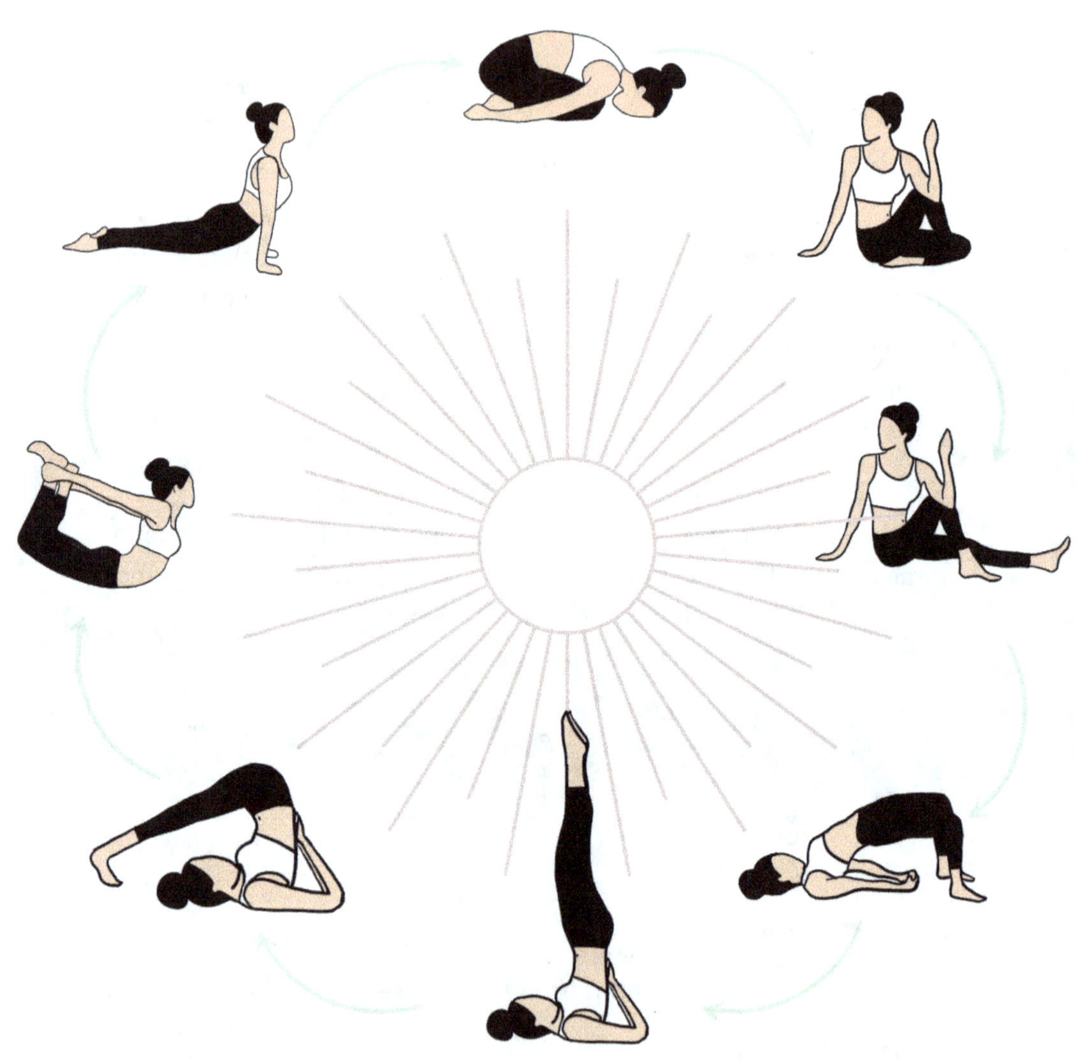

⭐ Hold the pose for 5-10 breaths

# DETOX FLOW B
## 8 YOGA POSES

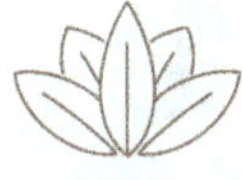

### Step 1:

Sit in Vajrasana pose or sit on your heels with your back straight.

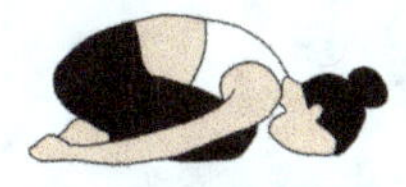

### ★ Step 2 :

Inhale, lengthen your spine. Exhale, bend forward, place your forehead on the mat.

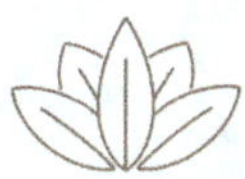

### Step 3 :

Inhale, bring your body up. Exhale, sit in Sukhasana pose or sit cross-legged. Bring your right knee up and place the right foot next to your left thigh.

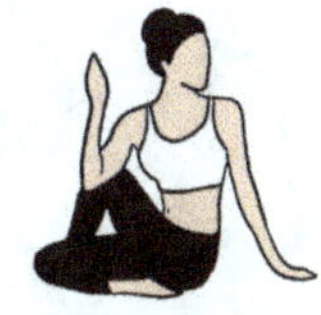

### ★ Step 6 :

Inhale, raise your arms up to shoulder level. Exhale, twist the body to the left. Right arm against left knee and left hand behind your back.

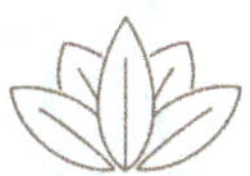

### Step 5 :

Inhale, back to the centre. Bring the right leg back and lift the left knee up. Left foot next to the right thigh.

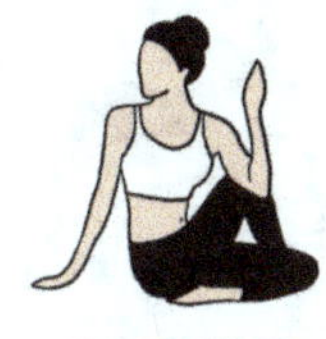

### ★ Step 4 :

Inhale, raise your arms up to shoulder level. Exhale, twist your body to your right. Left arm against right knee and right hand behind your back.

★ Hold the pose for 5-10 breaths

# DETOX FLOW B
## 8 YOGA POSES

### Step 7 :

Inhale, back to the centre. Exhale, sit in Dandasana pose or sit with your legs straight.

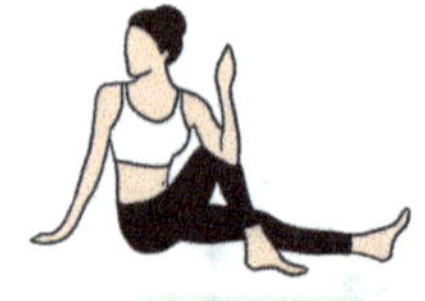

### ★ Step 8 :

Inhale, bring your right knee up, arms at shoulder level. Exhale, twist the body to the right. Left arm against right knee and right hand at the back.

### Step 9 :

Inhale, back to the centre. Exhale, right leg straight.

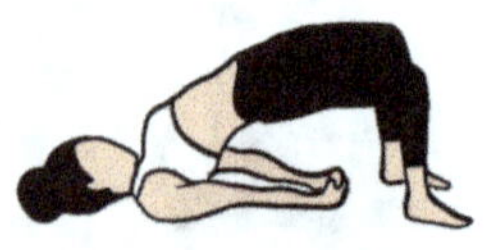

### ★ Step 12 :

Inhale, press your palms firmly on the mat and lift your hips up as high as possible. Your chin touching your chest; put your feet flat on the mat.

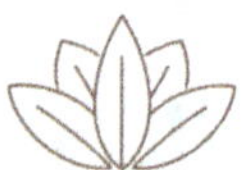

### Step 11 :

Inhale, back to the centre. Exhale, lay down on your back with your knees up.

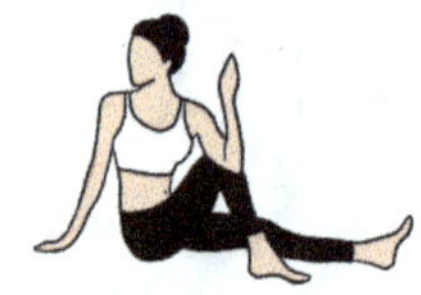

### ★ Step 10 :

Inhale, bring your left knee up, arms at shoulder level. Exhale, twist to the left. Right arm against left knee. Left hand at the back.

★ Hold the pose for 5-10 breaths

# DETOX FLOW B
## 8 YOGA POSES

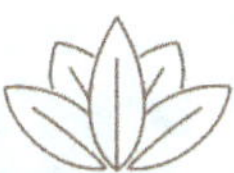

**Step 13:**

Exhale, lower your hips down on the mat.

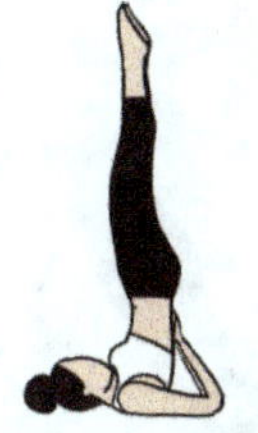

★ **Step 14 :**

Inhale, lift your legs and your hips up. Engage your core and your legs.

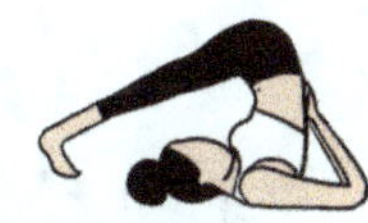

★ **Step 15 :**

Exhale, lower your legs down over your head and place your toes on the mat.

**Step 18 :**

Exhale, lower your legs and your chest down and release your hands from your ankles, your legs straight.

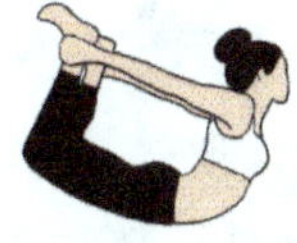

★ **Step 17 :**

Inhale, grab your ankles with your hands and slowly push your legs up while lengthening your front.

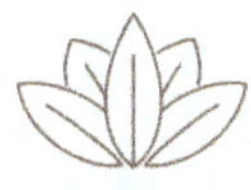

**Step 16 :**

Inhale, lift your legs up straight. Exhale, lower your legs down. Then lay down on your front.

★ **Step 19 :**

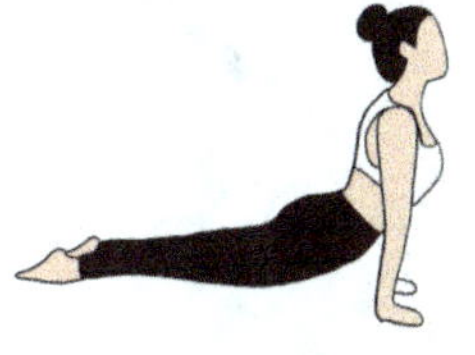

Place your palms next to your chest. Inhale, press your hands firmly on the mat and slide your body up with your arms straight.

REPEAT FROM
THE BEGINNING
TO FLOW MORE

★ Hold the pose for 5-10 breaths

# DETOX FLOW C

## 8 YOGA POSES

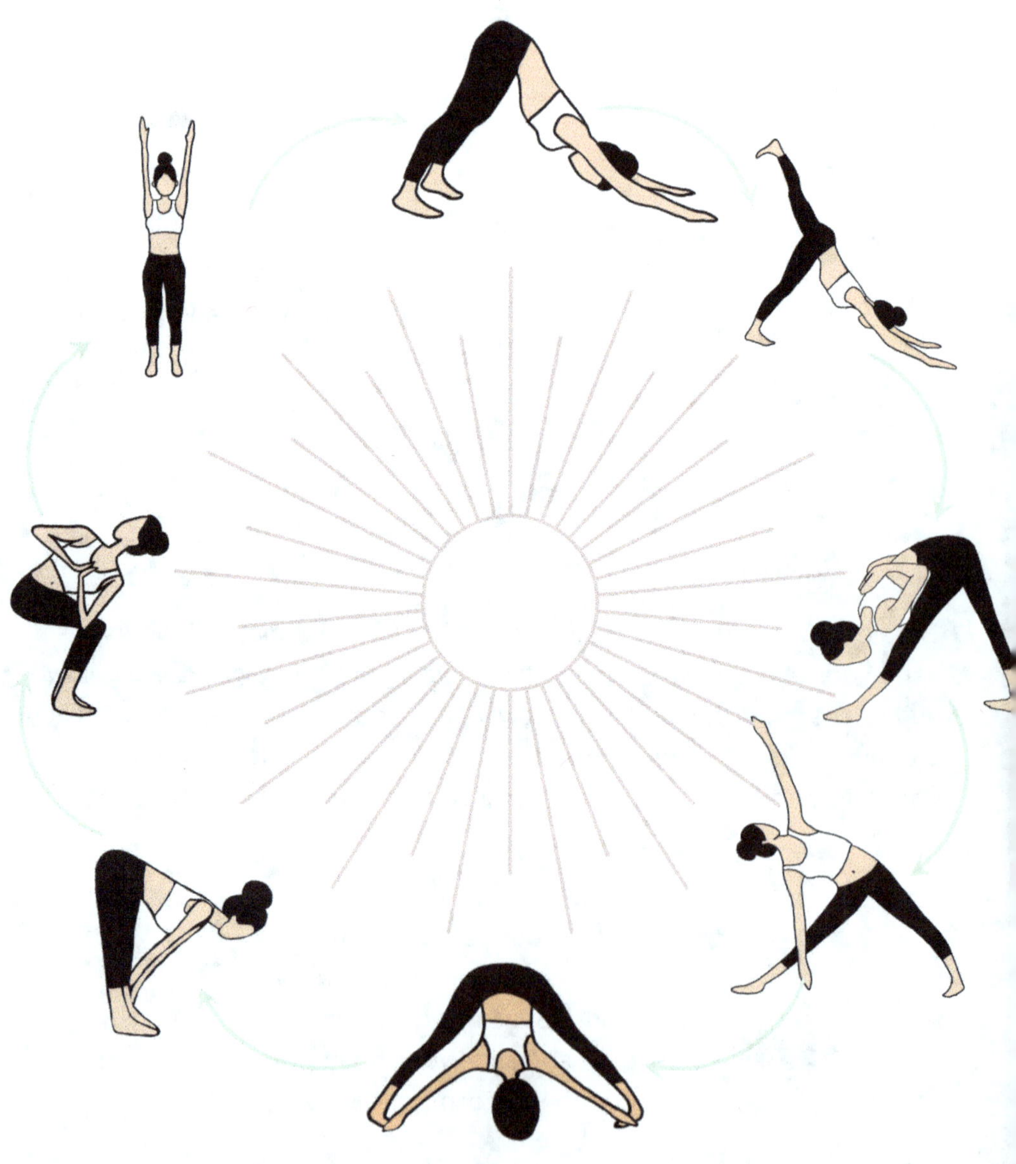

★ Hold the pose for 5-10 breaths

# DETOX FLOW C
## 8 YOGA POSES

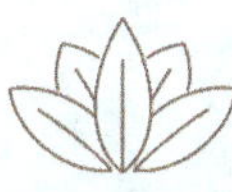

### Step 1:

Start in with table top position.

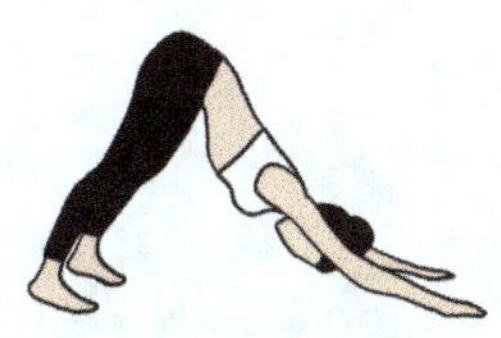

### Step 2 :

Inhale, press your palms firmly on the mat and lift your hips up. Exhale, push your hips toward the back.

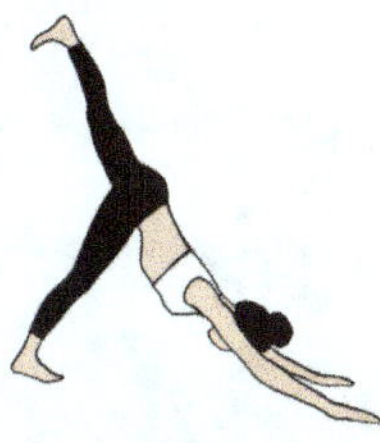

### Step 3 :

Inhale, lift your right leg up and push your hips toward the back.

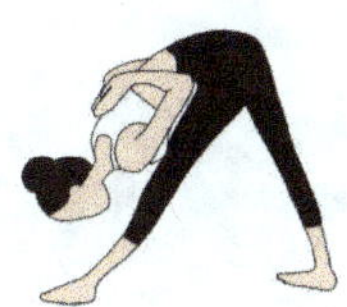

### Step 6 :

Inhale, bring your body up, hands touch behind your back. Exhale, bend forward with your legs straight.

### Step 5 :

Exhale, bring your left leg down. Inhale, right knee to your chest. Exhale, place your right foot in between your palms.

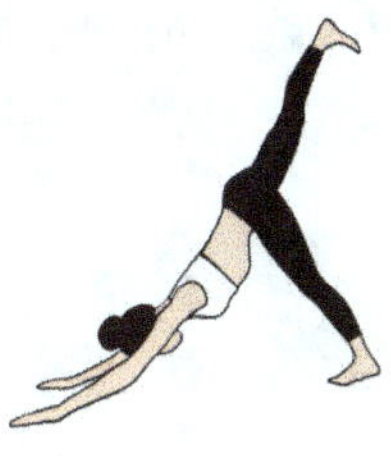

### Step 4 :

Exhale, bring your right leg down. Inhale, lift your left leg up and push your hips toward the back.

★ Hold the pose for 5-10 breaths

# DETOX FLOW C
## 8 YOGA POSES

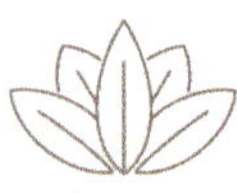

### Step 7:

Inhale, bring your body up. Exhale, hands at your waist. Adjust your left foot, pointing to the left, your hips are opened and aligned with the mat.

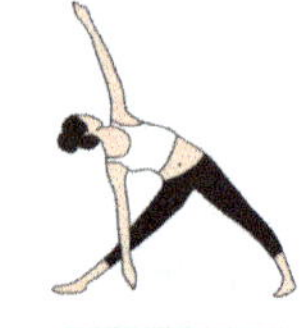

### ⭐ Step 8 :

Inhale, arms at shoulder level. Exhale, bend to the right, right hand on the mat and eyes fixed at left hand.

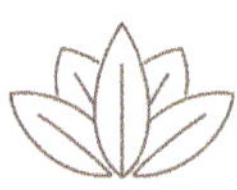

### Step 9 :

Inhale, bring your body up. Exhale, adjust your hips and your left foot pointing to the top of the mat. Replace right foot with left foot.

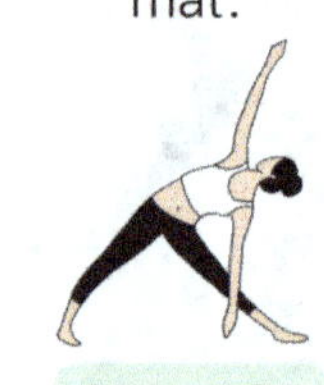

### ⭐ Step 12 :

Inhale, arms at shoulder level. Exhale, bend to the left, left hand on the mat and eyes gazing at right hand.

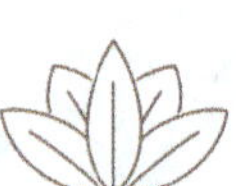

### Step 11:

Inhale, bring your body up. Exhale, hands at your waist. Adjust your right foot, pointing to the right, your hips are opened and aligned with the mat.

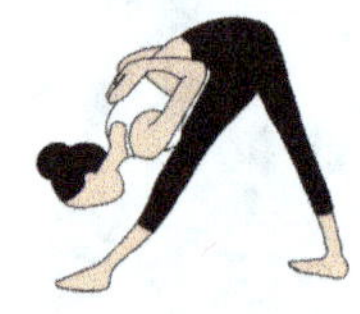

### ⭐ Step 10 :

Inhale, palms touch behind your back. Exhale, bend forward.

⭐ Hold the pose for 5-10 breaths

# DETOX FLOW C

## 8 YOGA POSES

### Step 13:

Inhale, bring your body up and hands at your waist. Adjust your feet, pointing to the right.

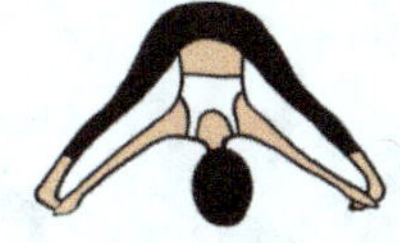

### ★ Step 14 :

Exhale, bend forward and slowly grab your big toes.

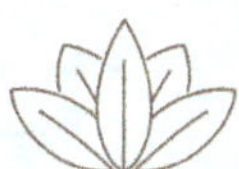

### Step 15 :

Inhale, bring your body up. Place your hands at your waist and your feet touch each other.

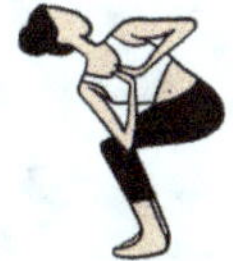

### ★ Step 18 :

Inhale, bring your body back to the centre. Exhale, twist your body to the left.

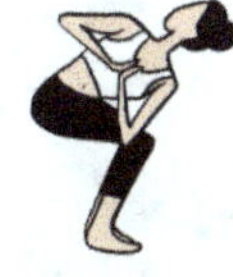

### ★ Step 17 :

Inhale, bring your body up, palms touching at your chest. Exhale, twist your body to the right.

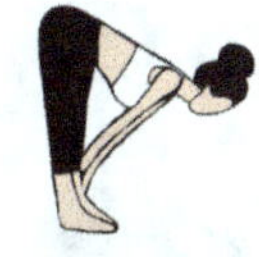

### ★ Step 16 :

Inhale, raise your palms up. Exhale, bend forward, palms on your legs or the mat.

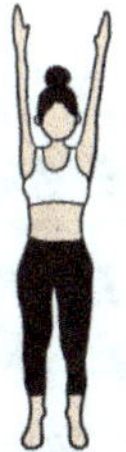

### ★ Step 19:

Inhale, raise your palms and your heels up. Exhale, heels on the mat and palms touching at your chest to end the flow.

**REPEAT FROM THE BEGINNING TO FLOW MORE**

★ Hold the pose for 5-10 breaths

# FULL DETOX FLOW
## 23 YOGA POSES

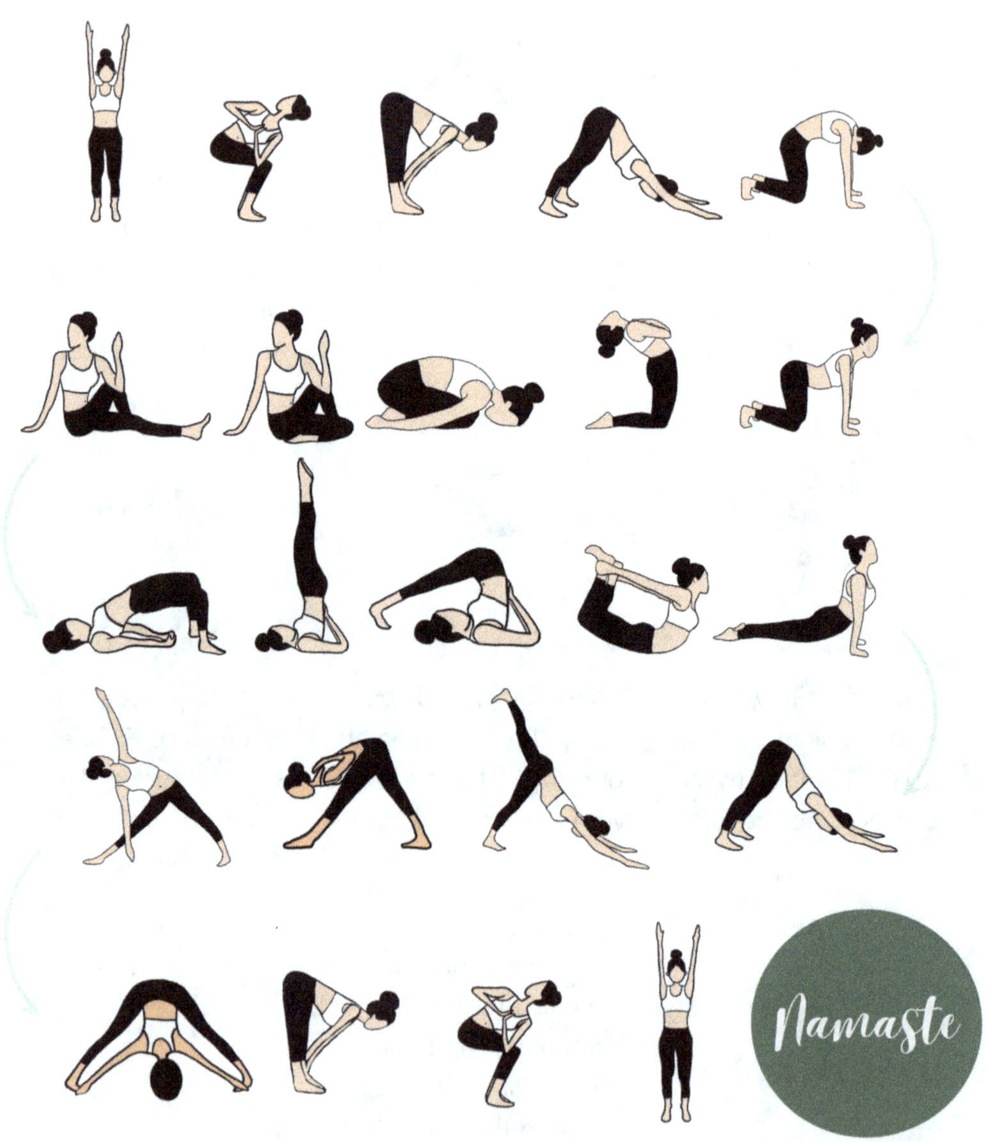


⭐ Hold the pose for 5-10 breaths

# FULL DETOX FLOW
## 23 YOGA POSES

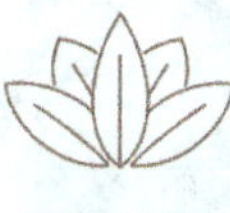

**Step 1:**

Stand tall, feet apart, legs, glutes and abs engaged.

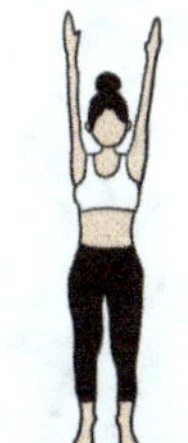

⭐ **Step 2 :**

Inhale, raise your palms and your heels up.

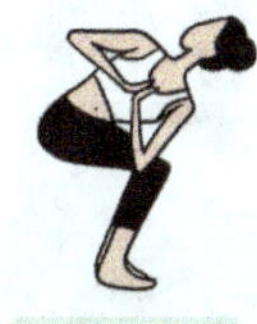

⭐ **Step 3 :**

Exhale, heels on the mat and bend your knees. Palms together at your chest, twist your spine to the right.

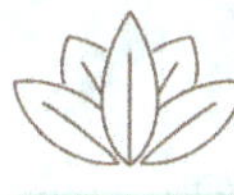

**Step 6 :**

Inhale, return your body to the centre and your legs straight.

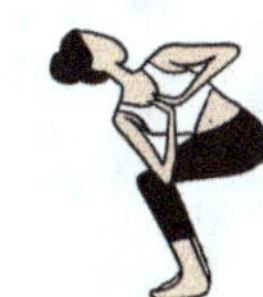

⭐ **Step 5 :**

Exhale, twist your body to the left.

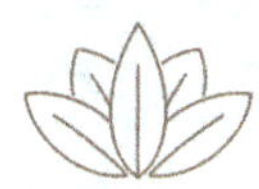

**Step 4 :**

Inhale, return your body to the centre.

⭐ Hold the pose for 5-10 breaths

# FULL DETOX FLOW

## 23 YOGA POSES

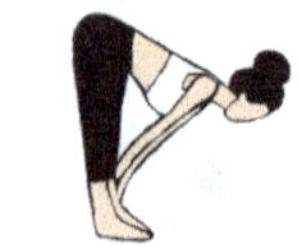

★ Step 7:

Exhale, bend forward, your fingers touch the mat or your palms on your legs.

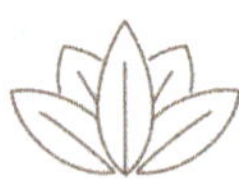

Step 8 :

Inhale, press your palms on the mat firmly, then step your legs to the back or jump to the back.

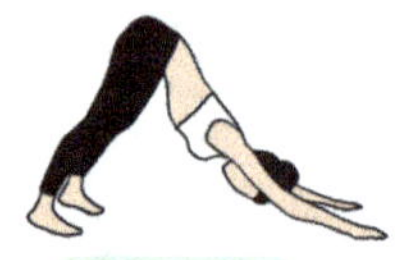

★ Step 9 :

Exhale, your feet on the mat, then push your hips toward the back.

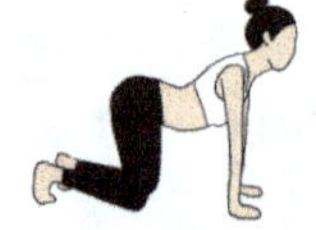

★ Step 12 :

Exhale, lower your belly down, lengthen your chest and your eyes look forward.

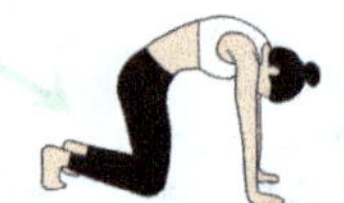

★ Step 11 :

Inhale, tuck your belly in, round your back, your chin touching your chest.

Step 10 :

Inhale, your eyes look forward. Exhale, place your knees down on the mat.

You can repeat the sequence 2-3 rounds

★ Hold the pose for 5-10 breaths

# FULL DETOX FLOW

## 23 YOGA POSES

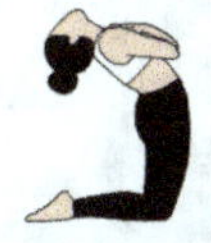

**Step 13:**

Inhale, stand on your knees and lengthen your chest toward the back. Exhale, push your hips forward.

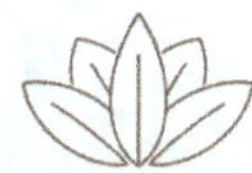

**Step 14 :**

Inhale, bring your body back to the centre.

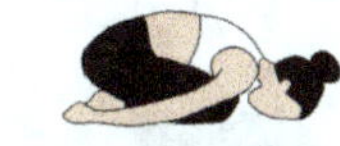

**Step 15 :**

Exhale, sit on your heels and bend forward. Your forehead is on the mat.

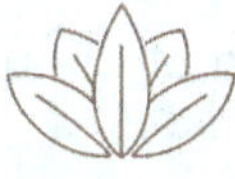

**Step 18 :**

Inhale, back to the centre. Bring the right leg back and lift the left knee up. Left foot next to the right thigh.

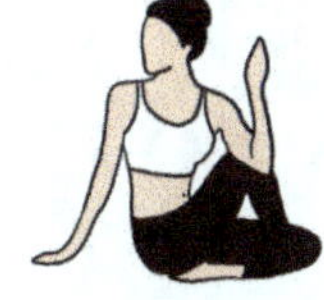

**Step 17 :**

Inhale, raise your arms up to shoulder level. Exhale, twist your body to your right. Left arm against right knee and right hand behind your back.

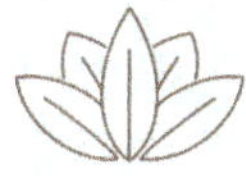

**Step 16 :**

Inhale, bring your body up. Exhale, sit in Sukhasana pose or cross-legged. Bring your right knee up and place the right foot next to your left thigh.

★ Hold the pose for 5-10 breaths

# FULL DETOX FLOW

## 23 YOGA POSES

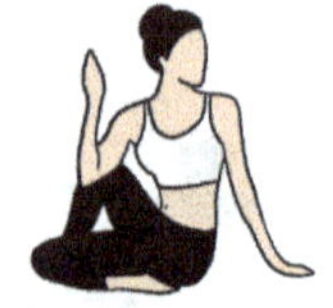

**Step 19 :**

Inhale, raise your arms up to shoulder level. Exhale, twist the body to the left. Right arm against left knee and left hand behind your back.

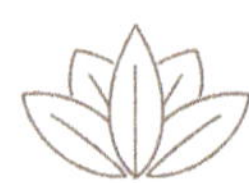

**Step 20 :**

Inhale, back to the centre. Exhale, sit in Dandasana pose or sit with your legs straight.

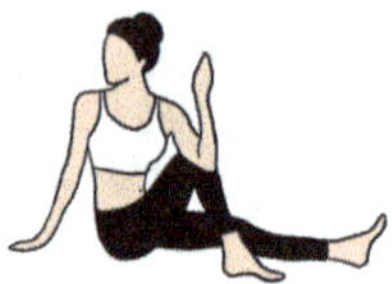

**Step 21 :**

Inhale, bring your right knee up, arms at shoulder level. Exhale, twist the body to the right. Left arm against right knee and right hand at the back.

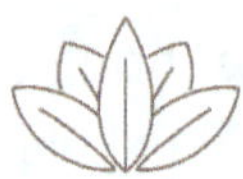

**Step 24 :**

Inhale, back to the centre. Exhale, lay down on your back with your knees up.

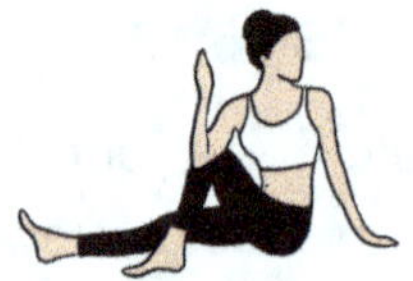

**Step 23 :**

Inhale, bring left knee up, arms at shoulder level. Exhale, twist to the left. Right arm against left knee. Left hand at the back.

**Step 22 :**

Inhale, back to the centre. Exhale, right leg straight.

★ Hold the pose for 5-10 breaths

# FULL DETOX FLOW
## 23 YOGA POSES

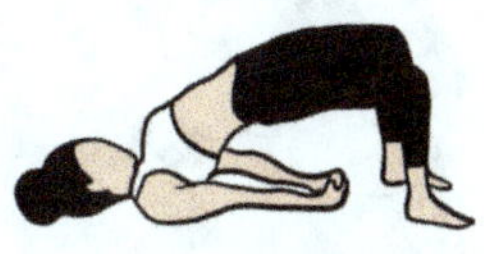

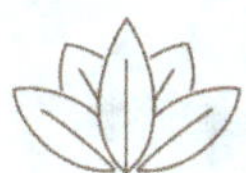

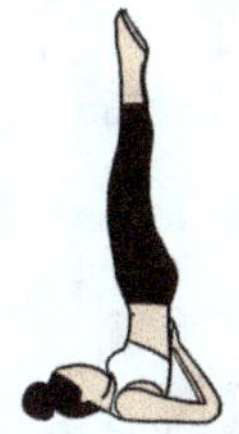

**Step 25 :**

Inhale, press your palms firmly on the mat, lift your hips up as high as possible. Your chin touching your chest your feet flat on the mat.

**Step 26 :**

Exhale, lower your hips down on the mat.

**Step 27 :**

Inhale, lift your legs and your hips up. Engage your core and your legs.

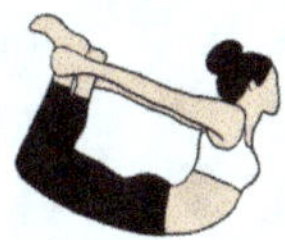

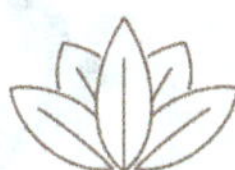

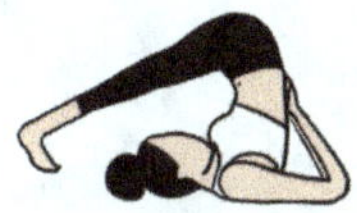

**Step 30 :**

Inhale, grab your ankles with your hands and slowly push your legs up while lengthening your front.

**Step 29 :**

Inhale, lift your legs up straight. Exhale, lower your legs down. Then lay down on your front.

**Step 28 :**

Exhale, lower your legs down over your head and place your toes on the mat.

★ Hold the pose for 5-10 breaths

# FULL DETOX FLOW
## 23 YOGA POSES

### Step 31 :

Exhale, lower your legs
and your chest down
and release your hands
from your ankles. Your
legs are straight.

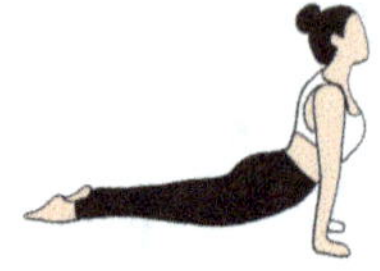

### ★ Step 32 :

Place your palms next
to your chest. Inhale,
press your hands firmly
on the mat and slide
your body up keeping
your arms straight.

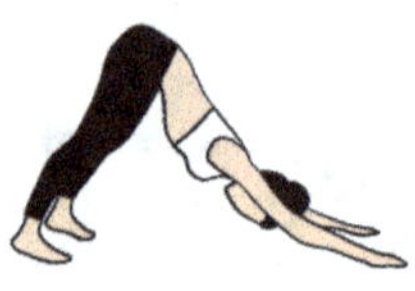

### ★ Step 33 :

Inhale, lift your hips
up. Exhale, push your
hips toward the back.

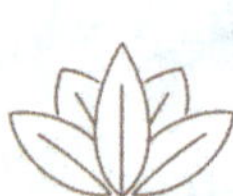

### Step 36 :

Exhale, bring your left
leg down. Inhale, right
knee to your chest.
Exhale, place right foot
in between your palms.

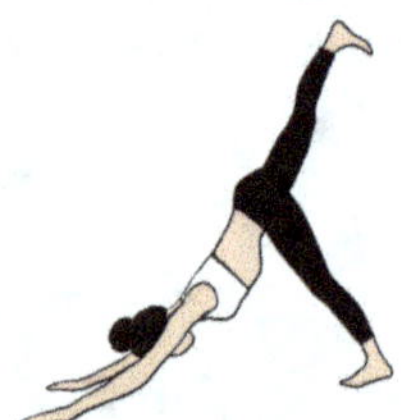

### ★ Step 35 :

Exhale, bring your
right leg down. Inhale,
lift your left leg up
and push your hips
toward the back.

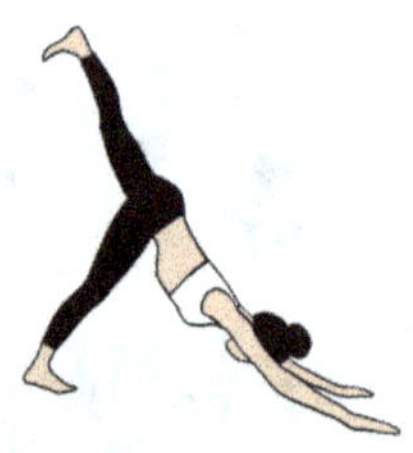

### ★ Step 34 :

Inhale, lift your right
leg up and push your
hips toward the back.

★ Hold the pose for 5-10 breaths

# FULL DETOX FLOW
## 23 YOGA POSES

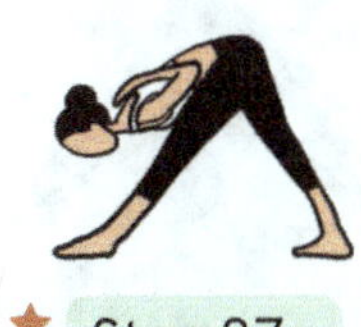

**Step 37 :**

Inhale, bring your body up, hands touching each other behind your back. Exhale, bend forward with your legs straight.

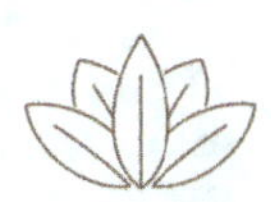

**Step 38 :**

Inhale, bring your body up. Exhale, hands at your waist. Adjust your left foot to point to the left, your hips are open and aligned with the mat.

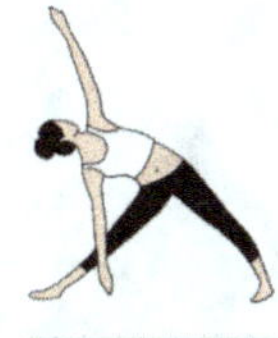

**Step 39 :**

Inhale, arms at shoulder level. Exhale, bend to the right, right hand on the mat and eyes gazing at left hand.

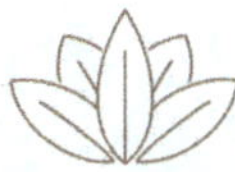

**Step 42 :**

Inhale, bring your body up. Exhale, hands at your waist. Adjust your right foot to point to the right, your hips are open and aligned with the mat.

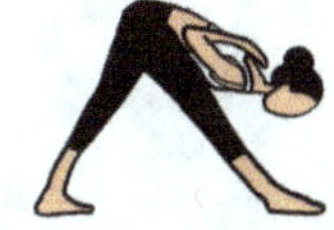

**Step 41 :**

Inhale, palms touching each other behind your back. Exhale, bend forward.

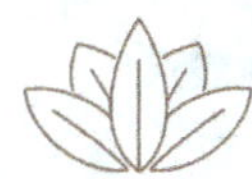

**Step 40 :**

Inhale, bring your body up. Exhale, adjust your hips and your left foot pointing to the top of the mat. Replace right foot with left foot.

⭐ Hold the pose for 5-10 breaths

# FULL DETOX FLOW

## 23 YOGA POSES

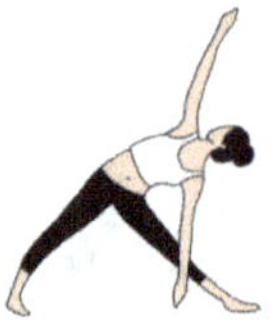



Inhale, arms at shoulder level. Exhale, bend to the left, left hand on the mat and eyes gazing at the right hand.

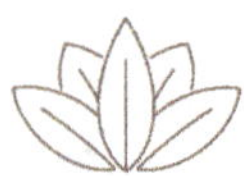



Inhale, bring your body up and hands at your waist. Adjust your feet to point to the right.

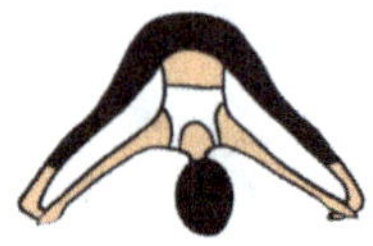



Exhale, bend forward and grab your big toes. Your eyes look to the back.

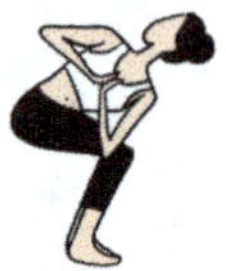



Inhale, bring your body up, palms touching at your chest. Exhale, twist your body to the right.

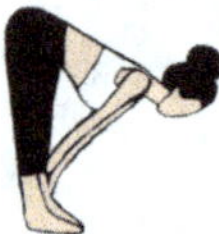



Inhale, raise your palms up. Exhale, bend forward, palms on your legs or the mat.

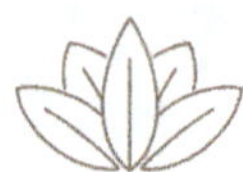



Inhale, bring your body up. Place your hands at your waist and your feet touch each other.

★ Hold the pose for 5-10 breaths

# FULL DETOX FLOW
## 23 YOGA POSES

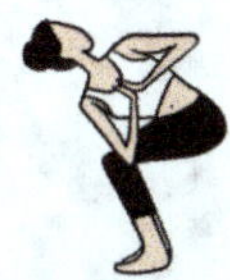

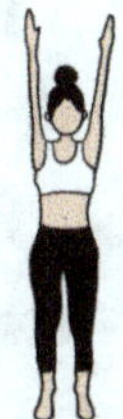

★ Step 49 :

Inhale, bring your
body back to the
centre. Exhale, twist
your body to the left.

★ Step 50 :

Inhale, raise your palms
and your heels up. Exhale,
heels on the mat and
palms touching at your
chest to end the flow.

★ Hold the pose for 5-10 breaths

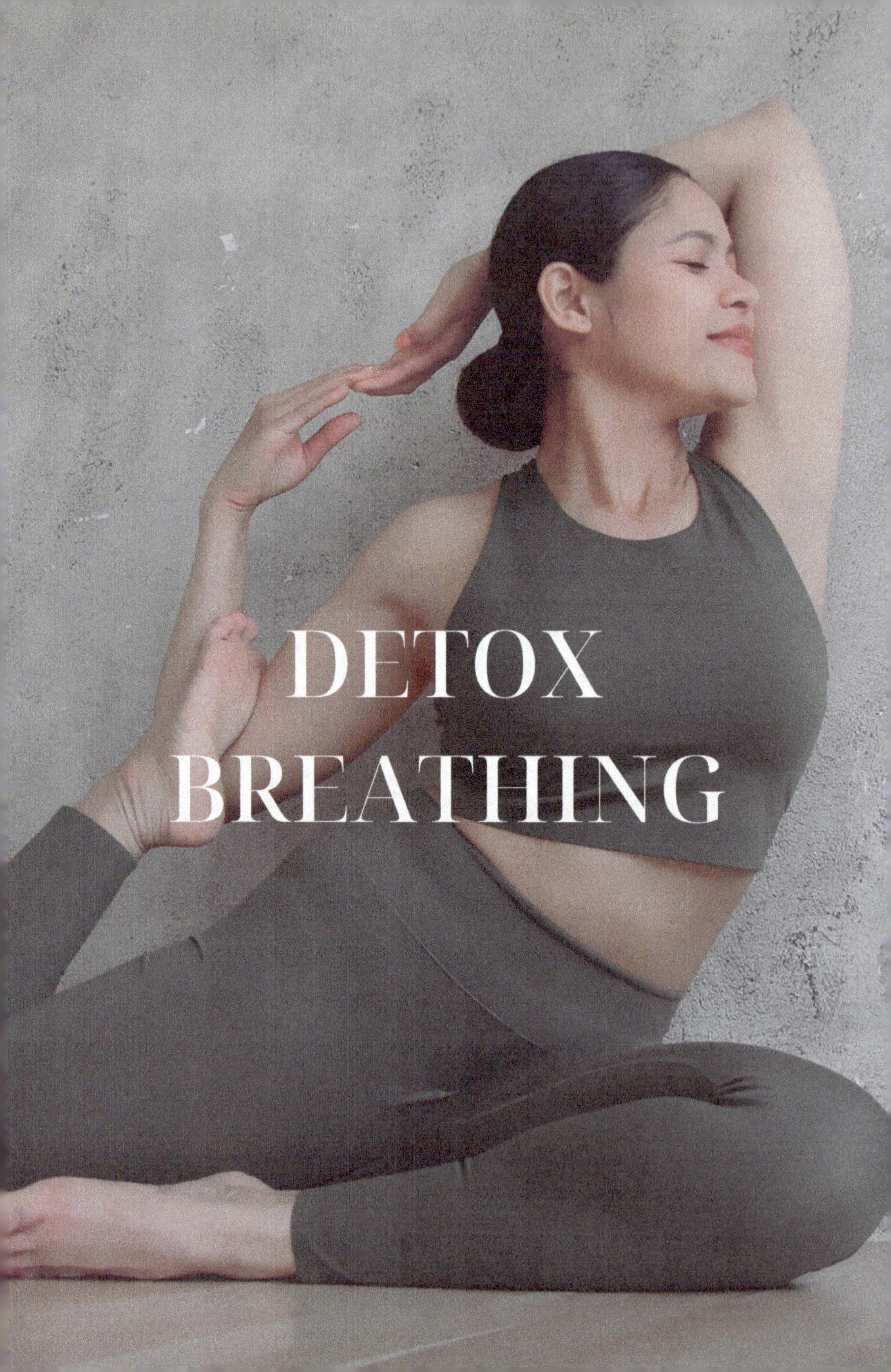

# DETOX BREATHING

# ...athing exercise to DETOX

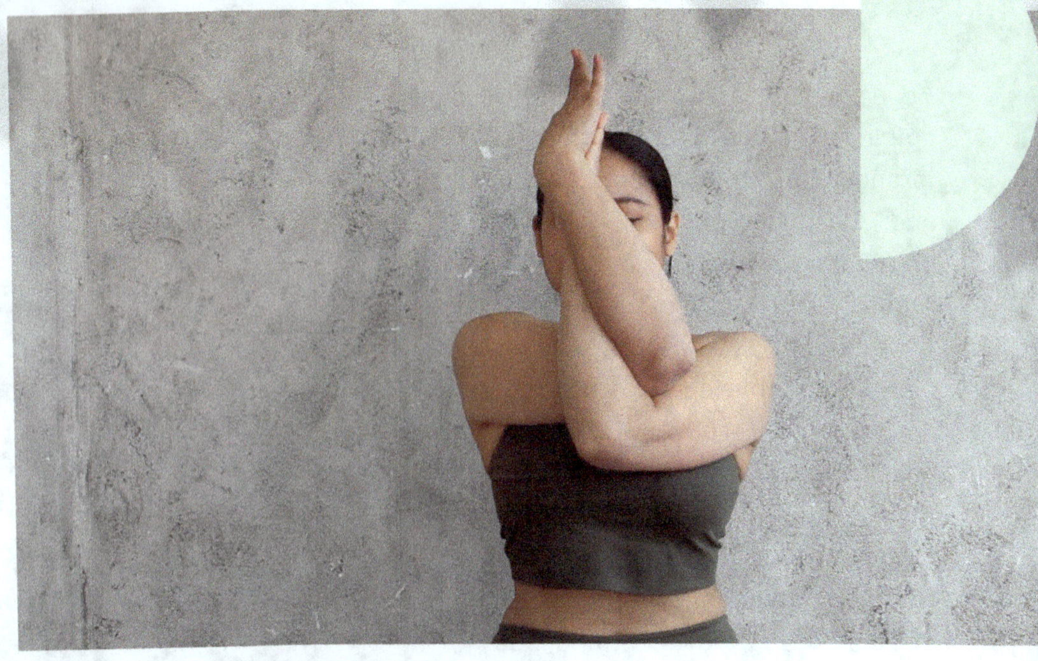

Getting oxygen in and releasing carbon dioxide from the body is the primary purpose of breathing. We can improve the respiratory function through proper deep breaths thus effectively getting air into all cells and helping lungs to improve the ability to remove toxins and gases. Each exhale from the body helps activating the parasympathetic system which keeps the body calm and relaxed. When the body is calm and relaxed the digestive/excretory system can function efficiently.

# Breath-work to DETOX

Yoga and Ayurveda have employed breathing techniques (pranayama) to maintain, balance and restore physical, mental, emotional, and spiritual health for thousands of years.

It results in several physiological benefits, achieved through the control of respiration. Ancient yogis have detailed different types of rhythmic deep breathing techniques and each of these breathing techniques has specific effects on the mind-body continuum.

The breathing techniques that we will use to detox our body in this book are as follows:
  1. Sama Vritti Breathing
  2. Ujjayi Breathing
  3. Kapalabhati Breathing
  4. Bhastrika Breathing

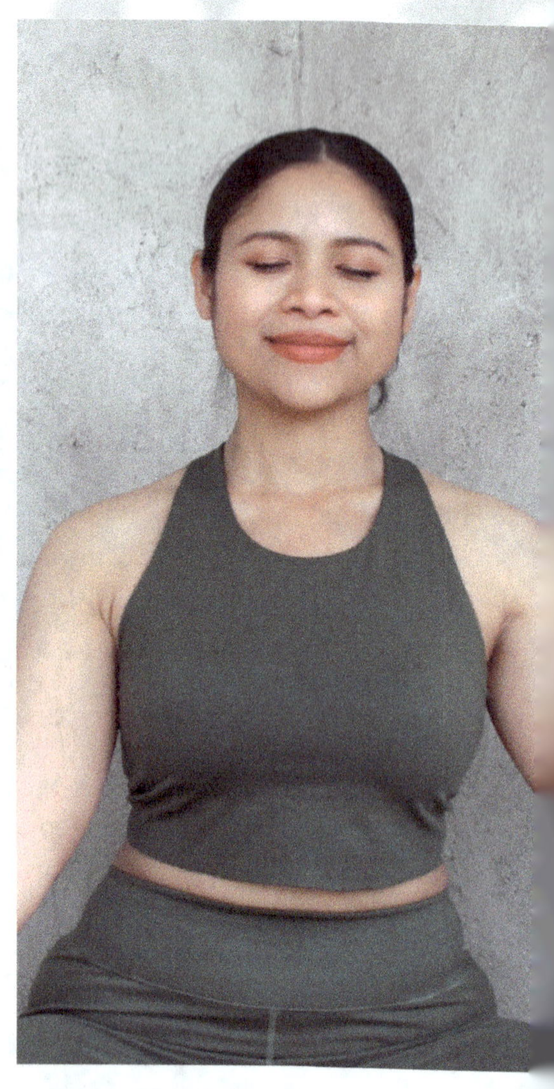

# Sama Vritti Pranayama
## BOX BREATHING

Sama Vritti Pranayama or Box Breathing is an equal breathing technique that uses a set of length of equal inhalations, exhalations and Kumbhaka or breath retention.

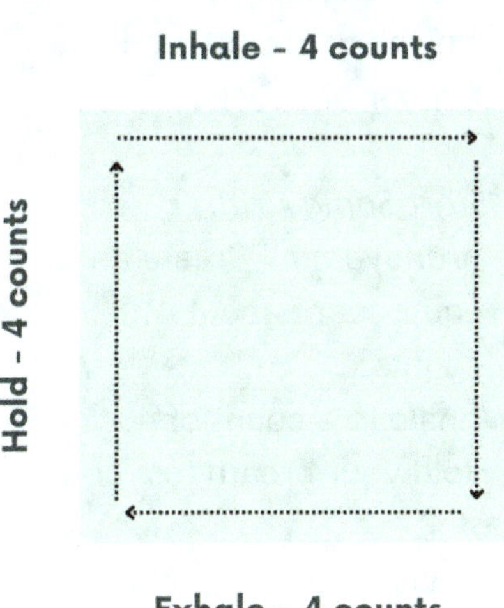



## Benefits of this pranayama:

The main benefits of this pranayama are to equalise, harmonise and balance the prana flowing through the nadis energy or energy channel. With the practice of Kumbhaka or breath retention, not only does this pranayama help calming the mind, reducing mental stress and worry, it also helps lungs to remove toxin from the system.

# Sama Vritti Pranayama
## BOX BREATHING

## How to practice:

1. *Find a comfortable position* - Start by finding the most comfortable position. It can be sitting in Sukhasana pose or lying down in Savasana pose with or without raising your knees. Make sure to relax your body and do not hold any tensions.

2. *Find your rhythm* - With the pranayama or yogic breathing slowly take a deep inhale and long exhale through your nose and try to slow and deepen your breath or count the number in your head for every breath you take. If you begin to struggle, then shorten the length and number of counts.

3. *Start Sama Vritti pranayama* - Create an equal set of about 4 counts.
- Inhale to a count of 4.
- Hold your breath to a count of 4.
- Exhale to a count of 4.
- Hold your breath to a count of 4.

# Sama Vritti Pranayama
**BOX BREATHING**

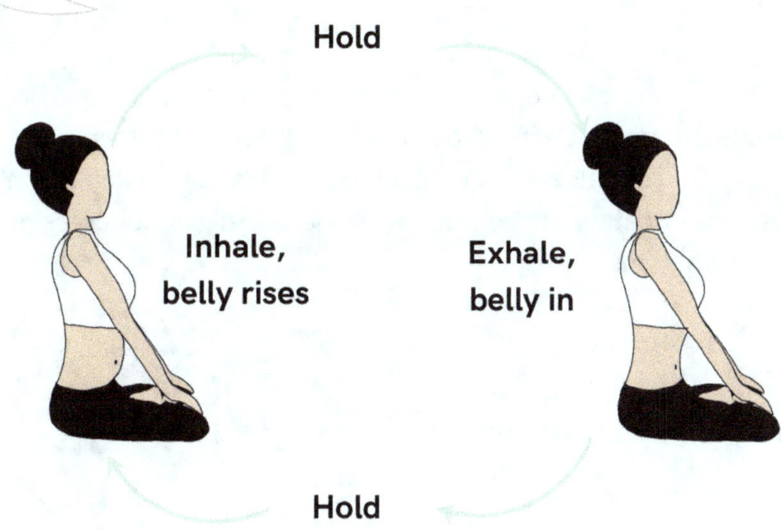


Repeat the flow for 2-6 rounds of breath. You can increase the duration to 10-30 breaths or a maximum of 10 minutes when you feel more comfortable with the practice.

## Cautions:

Pregnant women and people with blood pressure, lung, heart, eye or ear problems should avoid practice breath retention. If you feel dizzy or uncomfortable, stop box breathing and return to a normal relaxed breathing pattern.

# Ujjayi Pranayama
## OCEAN BREATHING

Ujjayi Pranayama or ocean breath is also known as Hissing Breath, Victorious Breath or Darth Vader Breath. Ujjayi is the best breathing technique for practicing Ashtanga Yoga. This breathing technique regulates the heating of the body with the air friction increasing the internal body temperature.

**Benefits of this pranayama:**

The main benefits of this breathing technique are to regulate the heat inside the body, massage the internal organs and stimulate the digestive system to encourage detoxification and decrease phlegm. This breathing technique also soothes the nervous system, calms the mind and slows down the heart rate and lowers blood pressure.

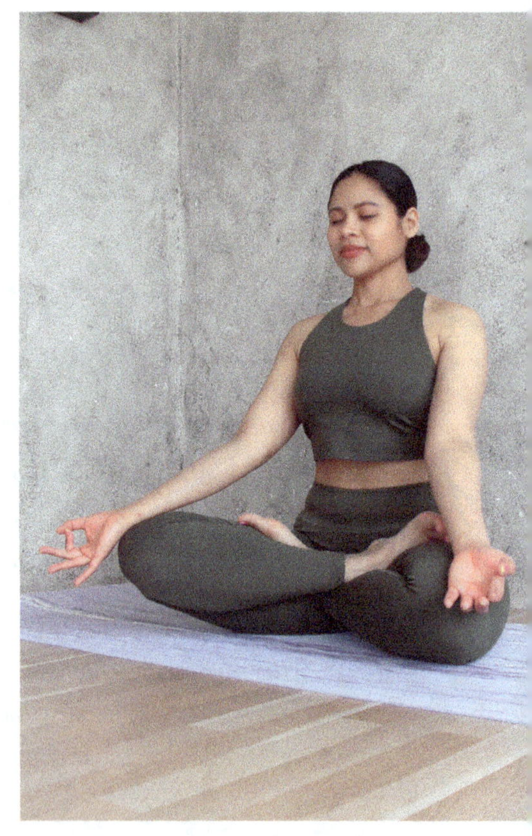

# Ujjayi Pranayama
## OCEAN BREATHING

**How to practice:**

1. *Find a comfortable position* - Start by finding the most comfortable position or in Sukhasana pose. Make sure your back is straight and your chest is opened.

2. *Constricting your throat* - Slightly constrict your throat or touch the palate with your tongue and feel the opening at the back of your throat below the epiglottis. Inhale and exhale through your nose with your mouth close.

You will hear a soft sound inside your throat akin to the gentle sound of the ocean.

3. *Engaging your belly* - Once you feel more comfortable, try engaging your belly and continue breathing through your nose like step 2. Try practicing up to 3 sets of 3 breaths each. You can slowly increase the set once you feel more comfortable.

# Ujjayi Pranayama
## OCEAN BREATHING

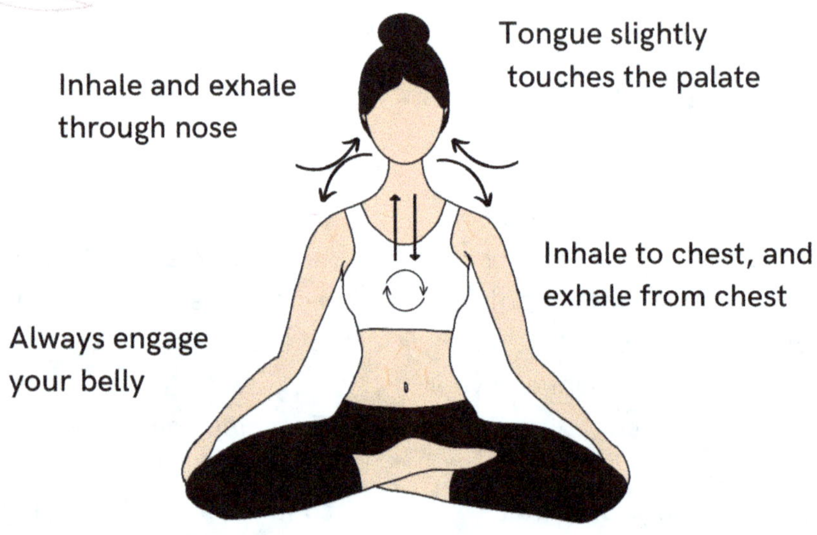


Try placing one of your hands on
your belly to make sure your abdomen stays engaged. Make
sure to not put too much pressure on your throat while
practicing.

## Cautions:

Pregnant women and people with heart condition, trauma and
anxiety should refrain from practicing. If you feel dizzy or
uncomfortable, stop and return to a normal relaxed
breathing pattern.

# Kapalabhati Pranayama
## SKULL-SHINING BREATHING

Kapalabhati or skull-shining breathing technique consists of alternating short, explosive exhales and slightly longer, passive inhales. Exhales are generated by powerful contractions of the lower belly (between the pubis and navel), which pushes air out of the lungs. Inhales are responses to the release of this contraction which sucks air back into the lungs.

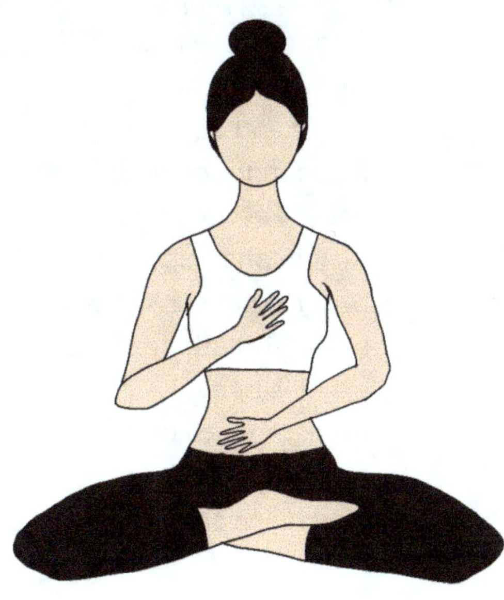

**Benefits of this pranayama:**

The key benefits of this pranayama are to clean or purify the lungs so they work at their best and strengthen the liver and kidneys. The Kapalabhati pranayama helps soothe sinus and asthma, improve blood circulation, digestion, and metabolism dramatically, energise your nerves, gain control over your mental strength, encourage hair growth, and detoxify your skin.

# Kapalabhati Pranayama
## SKULL-SHINING BREATHING

**How to practice:**

1. *Find a comfortable position* - Start by finding the most comfortable position. It can be sitting in Sukhasana pose or lying down in Savasana pose with or without slightly raising your knees. Make sure to relax your body and do not hold any tensions.

2. *Find your rhythm* - Start with few pranayama; deep inhales and long exhales. When you are ready, take a very deep inhale through your nose down to your belly, then push a short and strong exhale out from your belly by  pushing your navel to the spine then release it as if you were doing a belly pump.

3. *Start pumping* - Continue breathing as in step 2 but try to exhale faster and stronger and focus more on your belly. Feel your belly tuck in and push out in every exhale. Practice 3 sets of breathing, 5-10 exhales per set. Remember to breath normally few times after each set.

# Kapalabhati Pranayama
## SKULL-SHINING BREATHING

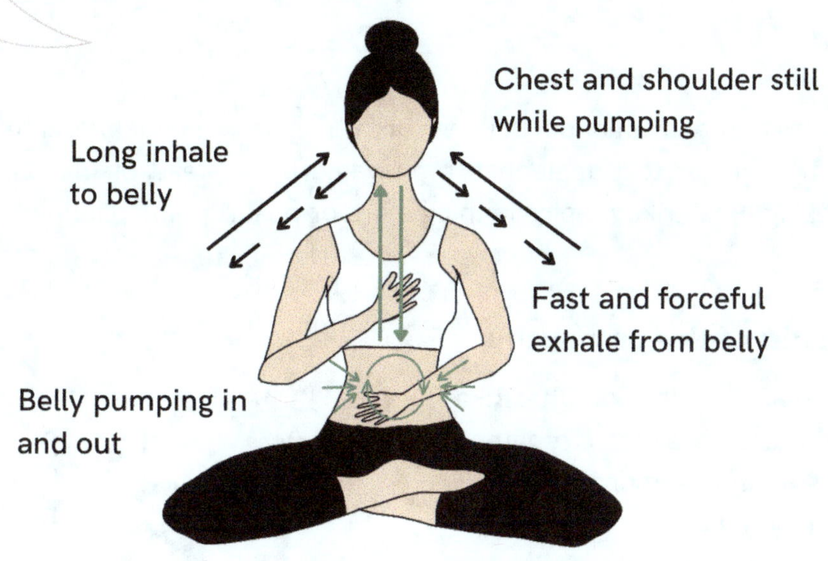


Try 10 -15 cycles with each cycle consisting of 10-15 explosive exhales after one long inhale. You can increase to up to 30 cycles once you feel more comfortable.

## Cautions:

Kapalabhati should not be practiced by pregnant or menstruating women and yogis with high or low blood pressure, heart disease, hernia, gastric ulcer, epilepsy, vertigo, migraine headaches, significant nosebleeds, detached retina, glaucoma, history of stroke; or by anyone who has undergone recent abdominal surgery.

# Bhastrika Pranayama
## BELLOWS BREATHING

Bhastrika Pranayama or Bellows Breathing is a heating breathing practice similar to Kapalabhati pranayama but instead of mimicking sneezing, Bhastrika mimics fanning a fire or post running panting.

### Benefits of this pranayama:

The main benefits of Bhastrika pranayama are to strengthen lungs and improve their capacity, increase oxygen in blood, remove toxin from the body and improve digestion. It cleanses and invigorates the liver, pancreas, and spleen, and helps freeing up nasal passages, sinuses, and chest of excess mucus. This breathing is good for people with depression and anxiety, and people who suffer from repetitive cough, flu, respiratory issues, allergies or breathlessness.

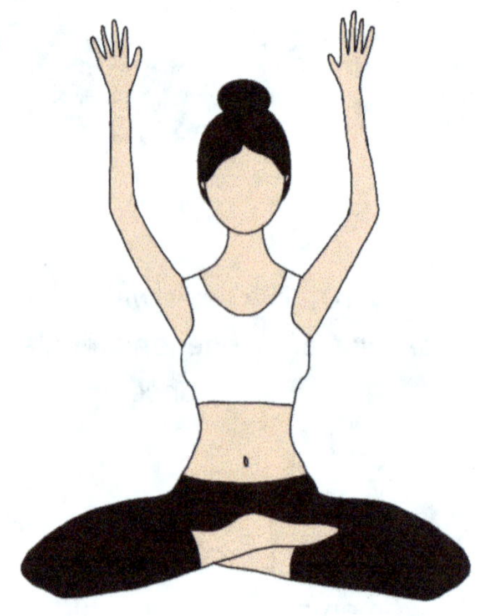

# Bhastrika Pranayama
**BELLOWS BREATHING**

## How to practice:

1. *Find a comfortable position* - Start by finding the most comfortable position. The recommended sitting position is Sukhasana pose or Vajrasana pose. Make sure to sit with your back straight.

2. *Find your rhythm* -  You can start by making a fist and fold your arms, placing them near your shoulders. Inhale deeply, raise your hands straight up and open your fists. Exhale slightly forcefully through your chest, bring your arms down next to your shoulders and close your fists.

Practice for few rounds until you understand the technique then you can increase the pace and intensity.

3. *Start Bhastrika pranayama* - Before you start the round make sure to take a few normal breaths. When you are ready, you can start with 3 sets of 10 reps. each. Remember to breath normally between sets.

# Bhastrika Pranayama
**BELLOWS BREATHING**

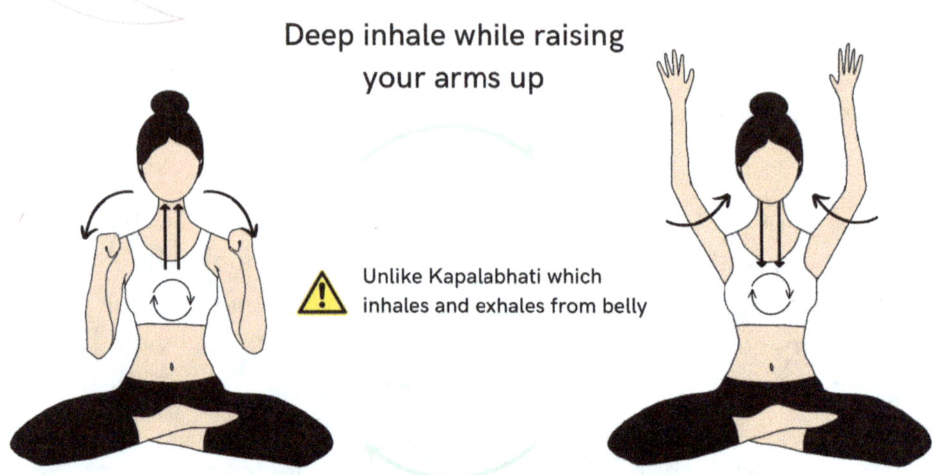



Making a fist and raising your arms help you to understand and practice easier. If you start feeling comfortable with this practice, you can rest your palms on your knees. You can also increase the reps from 10 breaths to up to 25 reps.

## Cautions:

Make sure to practice on an empty stomach. Pregnant women should not practice this breathing. People with high blood pressure, people who suffer from hypertension and panic disorders should be careful while practicing Bhastrika. If you feel dizzy or uncomfortable, stop and return to a normal relaxed breathing pattern.

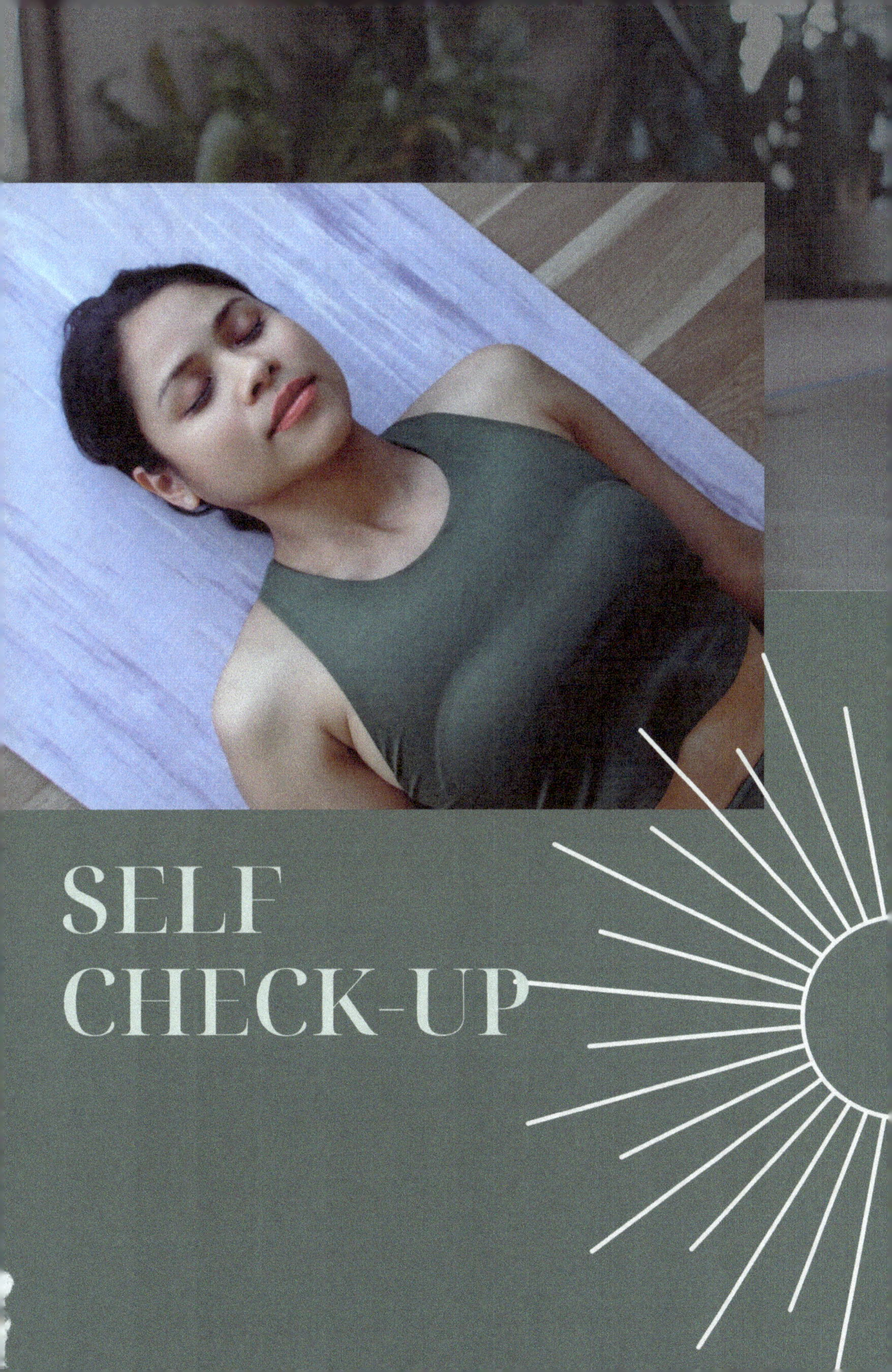
SELF
CHECK-UP

# DO I NEED TO DETOX?

*I HAVE BEEN EATING A LOT OF MEAT IN THE PAST FEW DAYS.*

- YES
- NO

*I DRINK ALCOHOLIC BEVERAGES ...*

- LESS THAN ONCE A WEEK
- 1-2 TIMES A WEEK
- 3-4 TIMES A WEEK
- MORE THAN 5 TIMES A WEEK

*I EAT PROCCESSED FOOD OR JUNK FOOD ...*

- LESS THAN ONCE A WEEK
- 1-2 TIMES A WEEK
- 3-4 TIMES A WEEK
- MORE THAN 5 TIMES A WEEK

I HAVE BAD BREATH EVEN AFTER I BRUSH MY TEETH.

- YES
- NO

## DO I NEED TO DETOX?

*I HAVE INSOMNIA OR FIND IT DIFFICULT TO SLEEP.*

- YES
- NO

*I USUALLY SLEEP BETWEEN 7-9 HOURS A NIGHT.*

- YES
- NO

*I DRINK AT LEAST 2 LITRES OF WATER A DAY.*

- YES
- NO

*I EAT BAKED GOODS OR SNACKS AT LEAST 3 TIMES A WEEK.*

- YES
- NO

*I DRINK FIZZY DRINKS OR SOFT DRINKS AT LEAST 3 TIMES A WEEK.*

- YES
- NO

# DO I NEED TO DETOX?

I HAVE BEEN CONSTIPATED FOR MORE THAN 2 DAYS.

- ⬤ ⬤ YES
- ⬤ NO

*I POOP AT LEAST ONCE A DAY.*

- ⬤ YES
- ⬤ NO

THIS IS THE SHADE OF MY STOOL.

- ⬤ YELLOW
- ⬤ BROWN
- ⬤ GREEN
- ⬤ ⬤ BLACK OR DARK BROWN

THIS IS THE SHAPE OF MY STOOL.

- ⬤ ⬤ NUT-SHAPED (SEPARATE HARD LUMPS)
- ⬤ ⬤ LUMPY SAUSAGE-SHAPED, HARD TO PASS
- ⬤ CRANKED SAUSAGE-SHAPED, EASY TO PASS
- ⬤ SMOOTH SAUSAGE-SHAPED OR SNAKE-SHAPED

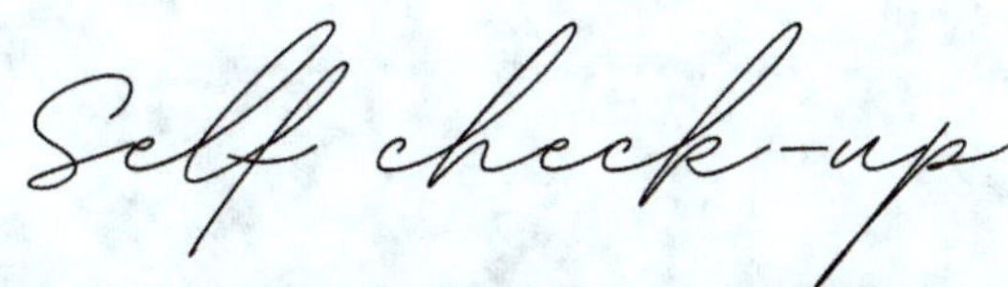



# DO I NEED TO DETOX?

**IF YOU TICKED MOSTLY RED ( ● ) YOU DEFINITELY NEED TO DETOX.**

If you have ticked a lot of red circles, don't be sad or worried. It is normal for everyone. The good thing is that now you know that your body needs your help to improve the systems and detox by readjusting your eating, drinking and sleeping habits. I prepared a 7-*day Detox Yoga plan* for you to help you boost up your system.

**IF YOU TICKED BOTH COLOURS EQUALLY THEN YOU CAN CHOOSE TO DETOX OR NOT TO**

If you have ticked both colours equally you are at a stage before it worsens. You can prevent your body from struggling to detoxify itself by following my *3-day Detox Yoga plan*. It is easy and it will make you and your body happy.

**IF YOU TICKED MOSTLY GREEN ( ● ) YOUR BODY IS DOING GREAT**

If you have ticked mostly green you can be happy and celebrate that you are taking good care of yourself. Your body is still able to detoxify and still keeps doing a great job. You don't need to do any detox, but you can improve your health by practicing *Yoga Flow A, B, C or Full Flow* wherever you want.

# DETOX YOGA
# PLANS

# $3$ DAYS DETOX YOGA

| | WARM UP | YOGA FLOW | BREATH | SVANASANA |
|---|---|---|---|---|
| DAY 1 | Ujjayi breathing 10 reps. x 3 sets | Practice Flow A & B x 3 sets | Use Ujjayi Pranayama during the flow | Box Breathing x10 reps. Savasana 10mins. |
| DAY 2 | Kapalabhati Pranayama 10 reps. x 3 sets | Practice Flow  B & C x 3 sets | Use Ujjayi Pranayama during the flow | Normal Prana x10 reps. Savasana 10mins. |
| DAY 3 | Kapalabhati Pranayama 10 reps. x 3 sets | Practice Full Flow (A,B,C) x 3 sets | Use Ujjayi Pranayama during the flow | Box Breathing x10 reps. Savasana 10mins. |

# $7$ DAYS DETOX YOGA

| | WARM UP | YOGA FLOW | BREATH | SVANASANA |
|---|---|---|---|---|
| **DAY 1** | Box Breathing 10 reps. x 3 sets | Practice Flow A  x 3 sets | Use normal pranayama during the flow | Normal Prana x10 reps. Savasana 10mins. |
| **DAY 2** | Box Breathing 15 reps. x 3 sets | Practice Flow  A x 3 sets | Use normal pranayama during the flow | Normal Prana x10 reps. Savasana 10mins. |
| **DAY 3** | Ujjayi breathing 10 reps. x 3 sets | Practice Flow B x 3 sets | Use Ujjayi Pranayama during the flow | Box Breathing x10 reps. Savasana 10mins. |
| **DAY 4** | Ujjayi breathing 15 reps. x 3 sets | Practice Flow B x 3 sets | Use Ujjayi Pranayama during the flow | Box Breathing x10 reps. Savasana 10mins. |
| **DAY 5** | Bhastrika Pranayama 10 reps. x 3 sets | Practice Flow C x 3 sets | Use Ujjayi Pranayama during the flow | Box Breathing x15 reps. Savasana 10mins. |
| **DAY 6** | Kapalabhati Pranayama 10 reps. x 3 sets | Practice Flow C x 3 sets | Use Ujjayi Pranayama during the flow | Box Breathing x15 reps. Savasana 10mins. |
| **DAY 7** | Bhastrika Pranayama 10 reps. x 2 sets Kapalabhati Pranayama 10 reps. x 2 sets | Practice Full Flow (A,B,C) x 1 set | Use Ujjayi Pranayama during the flow | 1Box Breathing x15 reps. Savasana 10mins. |

# DETOX YOGA WORKBOOK

# Daily Detox Tracker

S  M  T  W  T  F  S    DATE:

## Today's Affirmation:

## MY MEAL

- Breakfast :
- Snack :
- Lunch :
- Snack :
- Dinner :

### DETOX YOGA

Flow A   x   ............. sets

Flow B   x   ............. sets

Flow C   x   ............. sets

Full Flow   x   ............. sets

### HOURS OF SLEEP

Bedtime :

Wake time :

### DETOX BREATHING

- Box Breathing
- Ujjayi Breathing
- Kapalabathi Breathing
- Bhastrika Breathing

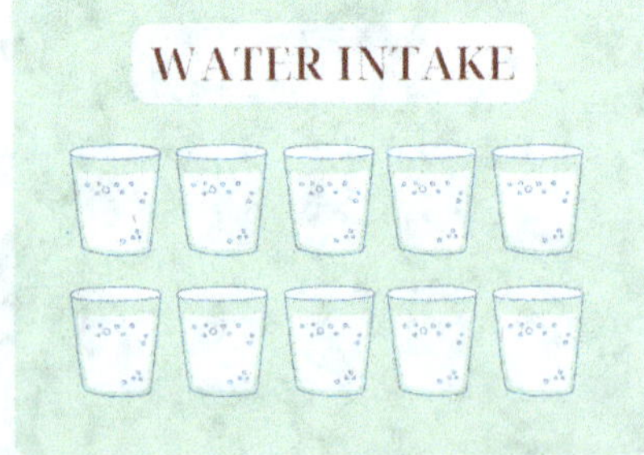

### WATER INTAKE

Toilet time :

# Daily Detox Checklist





**YES**

- [ ] Sleep 7-9 hours
- [ ] Do 5 minutes meditation
- [ ] Off screen 30 mins before bed
- [ ] Do Detox Breathing
- [ ] Do Detox Yoga
- [ ] Eat on time
- [ ] Eat 50% of veg in every meal
- [ ] Drink at least 2.5L of water
- [ ] Drink less coffee or tea
- [ ] Cook your own food
- [ ] Use less oil or butter to cook
- [ ] Have early dinner
- [ ] Eat a bit of fruits
- [ ] Walk at least 6,000 steps

**NO**

- [ ] Do not go to bed late
- [ ] Do not skip meal
- [ ] Do not eat red meat
- [ ] Do not eat processed food
- [ ] Do not snack on corn or potato crisps
- [ ] Do not eat deep fried food
- [ ] Do not go to bed with a full stomach
- [ ] Do not drink soft drinks
- [ ] Do not drink alcohol

S  M  T  W  T  T  S

DATE:

# Daily Evalution



DATE:

---

**How will you rate the following**

PHYSICAL

|  | Not at all | Low | Medium | High |
|---|---|---|---|---|
| I feel hungry | ○ | ○ | ○ | ○ |
| I feel good after practicing Detox Yoga | ○ | ○ | ○ | ○ |
| I have a good sleep | ○ | ○ | ○ | ○ |
| I feel comfortable with my stomach | ○ | ○ | ○ | ○ |
| I feel hydrated | ○ | ○ | ○ | ○ |

---

**How will you rate the following**

EMOTIONAL

|  | Not at all | Low | Medium | High |
|---|---|---|---|---|
| I am relaxed and calm | ○ | ○ | ○ | ○ |
| I am energised | ○ | ○ | ○ | ○ |
| I am happy with myself | ○ | ○ | ○ | ○ |
| I am motivated | ○ | ○ | ○ | ○ |

# Daily Detox Tracker



DATE:

## Today's Affirmation:

## MY MEAL

- Breakfast :
- Snack :
- Lunch :
- Snack :
- Dinner :

### DETOX YOGA

Flow A　x　............... sets

Flow B　x　............... sets

Flow C　x　............... sets

Full Flow　x　............... sets

### HOURS OF SLEEP

Bedtime :

Wake time :

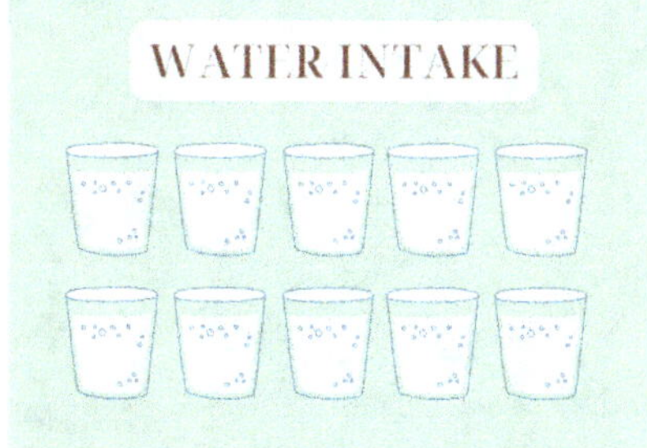

### WATER INTAKE

Toilet time :

### DETOX BREATHING

Box Breathing

Ujjayi Breathing

Kapalabathi Breathing

Bhastrika Breathing

# Daily Detox Checklist

**YES**

- [ ] Sleep 7-9 hours
- [ ] Do 5 minutes meditation
- [ ] Off screen 30 mins before bed
- [ ] Do Detox Breathing
- [ ] Do Detox Yoga
- [ ] Eat on time
- [ ] Eat 50% of veg in every meal
- [ ] Drink at least 2.5L of water
- [ ] Drink less coffee or tea
- [ ] Cook your own food
- [ ] Use less oil or butter to cook
- [ ] Have early dinner
- [ ] Eat a bit of fruits
- [ ] Walk at least 6,000 steps

**NO**

- [ ] Do not go to bed late
- [ ] Do not skip meal
- [ ] Do not eat red meat
- [ ] Do not eat processed food
- [ ] Do not snack on corn or potato crisps
- [ ] Do not eat deep fried food
- [ ] Do not go to bed with a full stomach
- [ ] Do not drink soft drinks
- [ ] Do not drink alcohol

S  M  T  W  T  F  S

DATE:

# Daily Evalution



DATE:

---

**How will you rate the following**

PHYSICAL

|  | Not at all | Low | Medium | High |
|---|---|---|---|---|
| I feel hungry | ○ | ○ | ○ | ○ |
| I feel good after practicing Detox Yoga | ○ | ○ | ○ | ○ |
| I have a good sleep | ○ | ○ | ○ | ○ |
| I feel comfortable with my stomach | ○ | ○ | ○ | ○ |
| I feel hydrated | ○ | ○ | ○ | ○ |

---

**How will you rate the following**

EMOTIONAL

|  | Not at all | Low | Medium | High |
|---|---|---|---|---|
| I am relaxed and calm | ○ | ○ | ○ | ○ |
| I am energised | ○ | ○ | ○ | ○ |
| I am happy with myself | ○ | ○ | ○ | ○ |
| I am motivated | ○ | ○ | ○ | ○ |

# Daily Detox Tracker

S  M  T  W  T  F  S          DATE:

Today's Affirmation:

## MY MEAL

Breakfast :

Snack :

Lunch :

Snack :

Dinner :

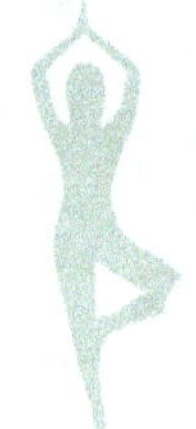

### DETOX YOGA

Flow A    x  ............... sets

Flow B    x  ............... sets

Flow C    x  ............... sets

Full Flow  x   ............... sets

### HOURS OF SLEEP

Bedtime :

Wake time :

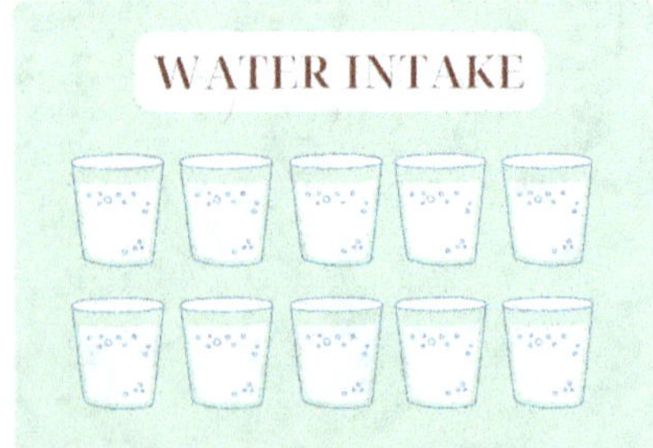



### DETOX BREATHING

Box Breathing

Ujjayi Breathing

Kapalabathi Breathing

Bhastrika Breathing

Toilet time :

# Daily Detox Checklist



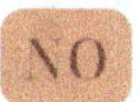


| YES | NO |
|---|---|
| ☐ Sleep 7-9 hours | ☐ Do not go to bed late |
| ☐ Do 5 minutes meditation | ☐ Do not skip meal |
| ☐ Off screen 30 mins before bed | ☐ Do not eat red meat |
| ☐ Do Detox Breathing | ☐ Do not eat processed food |
| ☐ Do Detox Yoga | ☐ Do not snack on corn or potato crisps |
| ☐ Eat on time | ☐ Do not eat deep fried food |
| ☐ Eat 50% of veg in every meal | ☐ Do not go to bed with a full stomach |
| ☐ Drink at least 2.5L of water | ☐ Do not drink soft drinks |
| ☐ Drink less coffee or tea | ☐ Do not drink alcohol |
| ☐ Cook your own food | |
| ☐ Use less oil or butter to cook | |
| ☐ Have early dinner | |
| ☐ Eat a bit of fruits | |
| ☐ Walk at least 6,000 steps | |

S M T W T F S

DATE:

# Daily Evalution



DATE:

---

**How will you rate the following**

**PHYSICAL**

| | Not at all | Low | Medium | High |
|---|---|---|---|---|
| I feel hungry | ○ | ○ | ○ | ○ |
| I feel good after practicing Detox Yoga | ○ | ○ | ○ | ○ |
| I have a good sleep | ○ | ○ | ○ | ○ |
| I feel comfortable with my stomach | ○ | ○ | ○ | ○ |
| I feel hydrated | ○ | ○ | ○ | ○ |

---

**How will you rate the following**

**EMOTIONAL**

| | Not at all | Low | Medium | High |
|---|---|---|---|---|
| I am relaxed and calm | ○ | ○ | ○ | ○ |
| I am energised | ○ | ○ | ○ | ○ |
| I am happy with myself | ○ | ○ | ○ | ○ |
| I am motivated | ○ | ○ | ○ | ○ |

# Daily Detox Tracker

( S ) ( M ) ( T ) ( W ) ( T ) ( F ) ( S )   DATE:

Today's Affirmation:

## MY MEAL

Breakfast :

Snack :

Lunch :

Snack :

Dinner :

## DETOX YOGA

Flow A   x   ............. sets

Flow B   x   ............. sets

Flow C   x   ............. sets

Full Flow   x   ............. sets

## HOURS OF SLEEP

Bedtime :
Wake time :

## DETOX BREATHING

Box Breathing

Ujjayi Breathing

Kapalabathi Breathing

Bhastrika Breathing

## WATER INTAKE

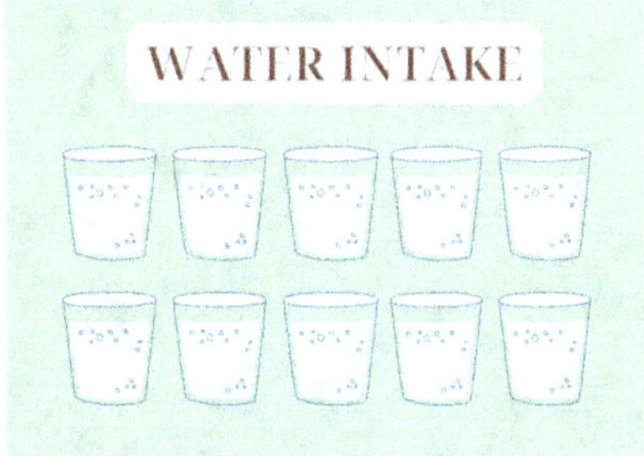

Toilet time :

# Daily Detox Checklist



**YES**

- ☐ Sleep 7-9 hours
- ☐ Do 5 minutes meditation
- ☐ Off screen 30 mins before bed
- ☐ Do Detox Breathing
- ☐ Do Detox Yoga
- ☐ Eat on time
- ☐ Eat 50% of veg in every meal
- ☐ Drink at least 2.5L of water
- ☐ Drink less coffee or tea
- ☐ Cook your own food
- ☐ Use less oil or butter to cook
- ☐ Have early dinner
- ☐ Eat a bit of fruits
- ☐ Walk at least 6,000 steps

**NO**

- ☐ Do not go to bed late
- ☐ Do not skip meal
- ☐ Do not eat red meat
- ☐ Do not eat processed food
- ☐ Do not snack on corn or potato crisps
- ☐ Do not eat deep fried food
- ☐ Do not go to bed with a full stomach
- ☐ Do not drink soft drinks
- ☐ Do not drink alcohol

S M T W T F S

DATE:

# Daily Evalution

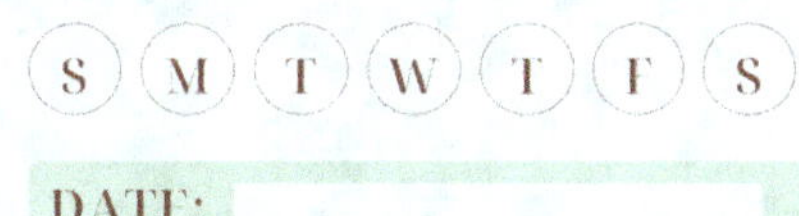



DATE:

---

**How will you rate the following**

PHYSICAL

| | Not at all | Low | Medium | High |
|---|---|---|---|---|
| I feel hungry | ○ | ○ | ○ | ○ |
| I feel good after practicing Detox Yoga | ○ | ○ | ○ | ○ |
| I have a good sleep | ○ | ○ | ○ | ○ |
| I feel comfortable with my stomach | ○ | ○ | ○ | ○ |
| I feel hydrated | ○ | ○ | ○ | ○ |

---

**How will you rate the following**

EMOTIONAL

| | Not at all | Low | Medium | High |
|---|---|---|---|---|
| I am relaxed and calm | ○ | ○ | ○ | ○ |
| I am energised | ○ | ○ | ○ | ○ |
| I am happy with myself | ○ | ○ | ○ | ○ |
| I am motivated | ○ | ○ | ○ | ○ |

# Daily Detox Tracker

S  M  T  W  T  F  S        DATE:

## Today's Affirmation:

## MY MEAL

Breakfast :

Snack :

Lunch :

Snack :

Dinner :

### DETOX YOGA

Flow A   x   ............. sets

Flow B   x   ............. sets

Flow C   x   ............. sets

Full Flow  x   ............. sets

## HOURS OF SLEEP

Bedtime :
Wake time :

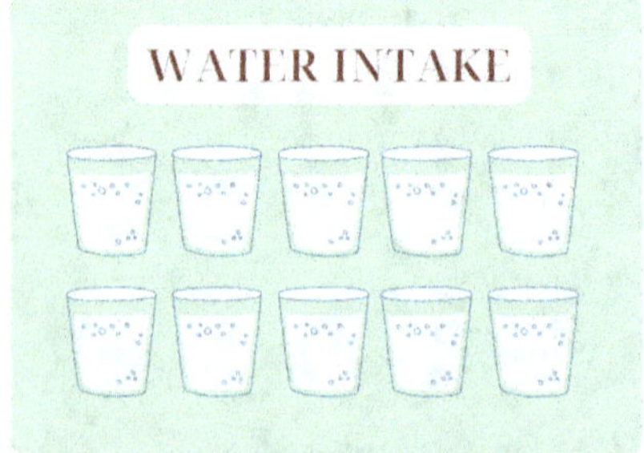

### WATER INTAKE

Toilet time :

### DETOX BREATHING

Box Breathing

Ujjayi Breathing

Kapalabathi Breathing

Bhastrika Breathing

# Daily Detox Checklist

YES 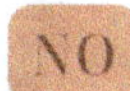 NO

**YES**

- ☐ Sleep 7-9 hours
- ☐ Do 5 minutes meditation
- ☐ Off screen 30 mins before bed
- ☐ Do Detox Breathing
- ☐ Do Detox Yoga
- ☐ Eat on time
- ☐ Eat 50% of veg in every meal
- ☐ Drink at least 2.5L of water
- ☐ Drink less coffee or tea
- ☐ Cook your own food
- ☐ Use less oil or butter to cook
- ☐ Have early dinner
- ☐ Eat a bit of fruits
- ☐ Walk at least 6,000 steps

**NO**

- ☐ Do not go to bed late
- ☐ Do not skip meal
- ☐ Do not eat red meat
- ☐ Do not eat processed food
- ☐ Do not snack on corn or potato crisps
- ☐ Do not eat deep fried food
- ☐ Do not go to bed with a full stomach
- ☐ Do not drink soft drinks
- ☐ Do not drink alcohol

S M T W T F S

DATE:

# Daily Evalution

S M T W T F S

DATE:

---

### PHYSICAL

**How will you rate the following**

|  | Not at all | Low | Medium | High |
|---|---|---|---|---|
| I feel hungry | ○ | ○ | ○ | ○ |
| I feel good after practicing Detox Yoga | ○ | ○ | ○ | ○ |
| I have a good sleep | ○ | ○ | ○ | ○ |
| I feel comfortable with my stomach | ○ | ○ | ○ | ○ |
| I feel hydrated | ○ | ○ | ○ | ○ |

### EMOTIONAL

**How will you rate the following**

|  | Not at all | Low | Medium | High |
|---|---|---|---|---|
| I am relaxed and calm | ○ | ○ | ○ | ○ |
| I am energised | ○ | ○ | ○ | ○ |
| I am happy with myself | ○ | ○ | ○ | ○ |
| I am motivated | ○ | ○ | ○ | ○ |

# Daily Detox Tracker

S  M  T  W  T  F  S    DATE:

## Today's Affirmation:

## MY MEAL

- Breakfast :
- Snack :
- Lunch :
- Snack :
- Dinner :

### DETOX YOGA

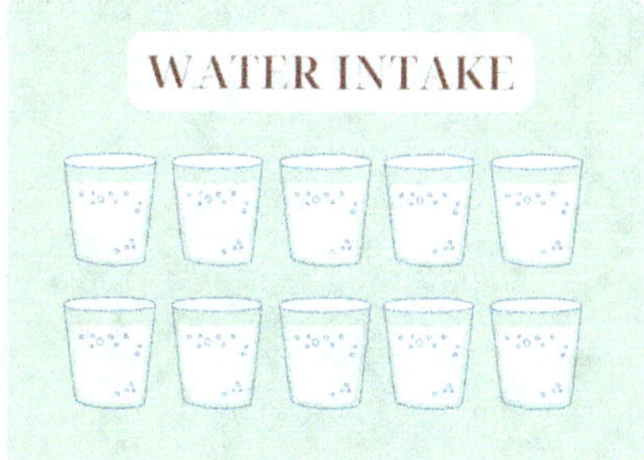

Flow A   x   ............. sets

Flow B   x   ............. sets

Flow C   x   ............. sets

Full Flow   x   ............. sets

### HOURS OF SLEEP

Bedtime :

Wake time :

### WATER INTAKE

Toilet time :

### DETOX BREATHING

Box Breathing

Ujjayi Breathing

Kapalabathi Breathing

Bhastrika Breathing

# Daily Detox Checklist



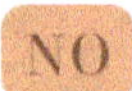


| YES | NO |
|---|---|
| ☐ Sleep 7-9 hours | ☐ Do not go to bed late |
| ☐ Do 5 minutes meditation | ☐ Do not skip meal |
| ☐ Off screen 30 mins before bed | ☐ Do not eat red meat |
| ☐ Do Detox Breathing | ☐ Do not eat processed food |
| ☐ Do Detox Yoga | ☐ Do not snack on corn or potato crisps |
| ☐ Eat on time | ☐ Do not eat deep fried food |
| ☐ Eat 50% of veg in every meal | ☐ Do not go to bed with a full stomach |
| ☐ Drink at least 2.5L of water | ☐ Do not drink soft drinks |
| ☐ Drink less coffee or tea | ☐ Do not drink alcohol |
| ☐ Cook your own food | |
| ☐ Use less oil or butter to cook | |
| ☐ Have early dinner | |
| ☐ Eat a bit of fruits | |
| ☐ Walk at least 6,000 steps | |

S  M  T  W  T  F  S

DATE:

# Daily Evalution

S  M  T  W  T  F  S

DATE:

---

## How will you rate the following

### PHYSICAL

|  | Not at all | Low | Medium | High |
|---|---|---|---|---|
| I feel hungry | ○ | ○ | ○ | ○ |
| I feel good after practicing Detox Yoga | ○ | ○ | ○ | ○ |
| I have a good sleep | ○ | ○ | ○ | ○ |
| I feel comfortable with my stomach | ○ | ○ | ○ | ○ |
| I feel hydrated | ○ | ○ | ○ | ○ |

---

## How will you rate the following

### EMOTIONAL

|  | Not at all | Low | Medium | High |
|---|---|---|---|---|
| I am relaxed and calm | ○ | ○ | ○ | ○ |
| I am energised | ○ | ○ | ○ | ○ |
| I am happy with myself | ○ | ○ | ○ | ○ |
| I am motivated | ○ | ○ | ○ | ○ |

# Daily Detox Tracker

( S ) ( M ) ( T ) ( W ) ( T ) ( F ) ( S )     DATE:

Today's Affirmation:

## MY MEAL

Breakfast :

Snack :

Lunch :

Snack :

Dinner :

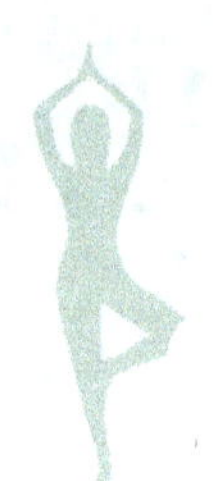

## DETOX YOGA

Flow A   x   ............. sets

Flow B   x   ............. sets

Flow C   x   ............. sets

Full Flow   x   ............. sets

## HOURS OF SLEEP

Bedtime :
Wake time :

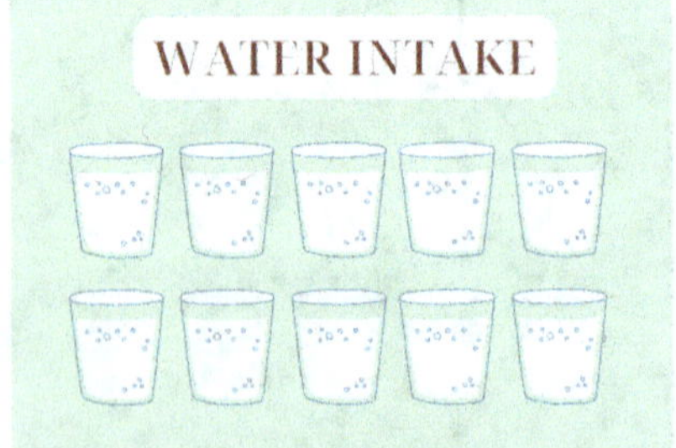


## DETOX BREATHING

Box Breathing

Ujjayi Breathing

Kapalabathi Breathing

Bhastrika Breathing

Toilet time :

# Daily Detox Checklist

YES        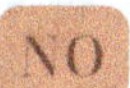NO

| YES | NO |
| --- | --- |
| ☐ Sleep 7-9 hours | ☐ Do not go to bed late |
| ☐ Do 5 minutes meditation | ☐ Do not skip meal |
| ☐ Off screen 30 mins before bed | ☐ Do not eat red meat |
| ☐ Do Detox Breathing | ☐ Do not eat processed food |
| ☐ Do Detox Yoga | ☐ Do not snack on corn or potato crisps |
| ☐ Eat on time | ☐ Do not eat deep fried food |
| ☐ Eat 50% of veg in every meal | ☐ Do not go to bed with a full stomach |
| ☐ Drink at least 2.5L of water | ☐ Do not drink soft drinks |
| ☐ Drink less coffee or tea | ☐ Do not drink alcohol |
| ☐ Cook your own food | |
| ☐ Use less oil or butter to cook | |
| ☐ Have early dinner | |
| ☐ Eat a bit of fruits | |
| ☐ Walk at least 6,000 steps | |

Ⓢ Ⓜ Ⓣ Ⓦ Ⓣ Ⓕ Ⓢ

DATE: __________

# Daily Evalution

S  M  T  W  T  F  S

DATE:

---

**How will you rate the following**

### PHYSICAL

| | Not at all | Low | Medium | High |
|---|---|---|---|---|
| I feel hungry | ○ | ○ | ○ | ○ |
| I feel good after practicing Detox Yoga | ○ | ○ | ○ | ○ |
| I have a good sleep | ○ | ○ | ○ | ○ |
| I feel comfortable with my stomach | ○ | ○ | ○ | ○ |
| I feel hydrated | ○ | ○ | ○ | ○ |

---

**How will you rate the following**

### EMOTIONAL

| | Not at all | Low | Medium | High |
|---|---|---|---|---|
| I am relaxed and calm | ○ | ○ | ○ | ○ |
| I am energised | ○ | ○ | ○ | ○ |
| I am happy with myself | ○ | ○ | ○ | ○ |
| I am motivated | ○ | ○ | ○ | ○ |

"Physical fitness is
the first requisite of
happiness."

– Joseph Pilates

# FAQs

### What is Yoga?

Yoga is a practice of body and mind through yoga asana and pranayama (breathing technique) which lead us to have mental peace and healthy body.

### Can I do Detox Yoga if I'm not flexible?

You don't need to be flexible to do yoga. On the other hand, practicing yoga makes you flexible. So, you can do Detox Yoga even though you are not flexible. Just do it at your own pace and enjoy the movement.

### When should I practice Detox Yoga?

The best time to practice Detox Yoga is in the morning after waking up and before breakfast. You can also practice during the day or in the evening, but make sure your stomach is empty or wait up for 3-4 hours after eating.

### Can I do Detox Yoga if I don't have a yoga background?

You definitely can do Detox Yoga even though you've never practiced yoga before. The instructions in the book are very simple and easy to follow.

### How to do Yogic breathing or normal pranayama?

You can practice by sitting in a comfortable position, your back straight; relax your body. Take a deep inhale through your nose, feel your belly rise and your rib cage expand. Exhale, your chest drops down and your belly pushes back in.

### Can I drink detox water during the programme?

Yes, you can drink detox water during the 3 days or 7 days Detox Yoga programme.

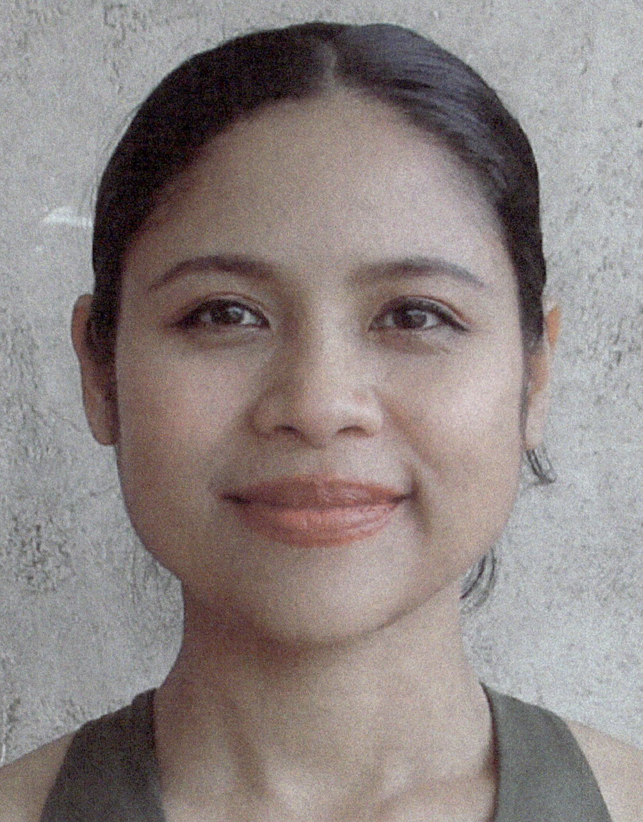

Hello dear reader,

thank you for having this book in your hands. I do hope that you find it useful and insightful.

I am a Thai yoga teacher  who completed a Yoga Teacher Training course in Bangkok, Thailand, but now living and teaching yoga in Paris, France.

I started writing this book in 2021. I try my best to make it easy to read, to understand, and most importantly easy to follow along.

If you like my book and would like to discover more about yoga, visit amber-yoga.com or get in touch on Instagram @Amber.ynwl

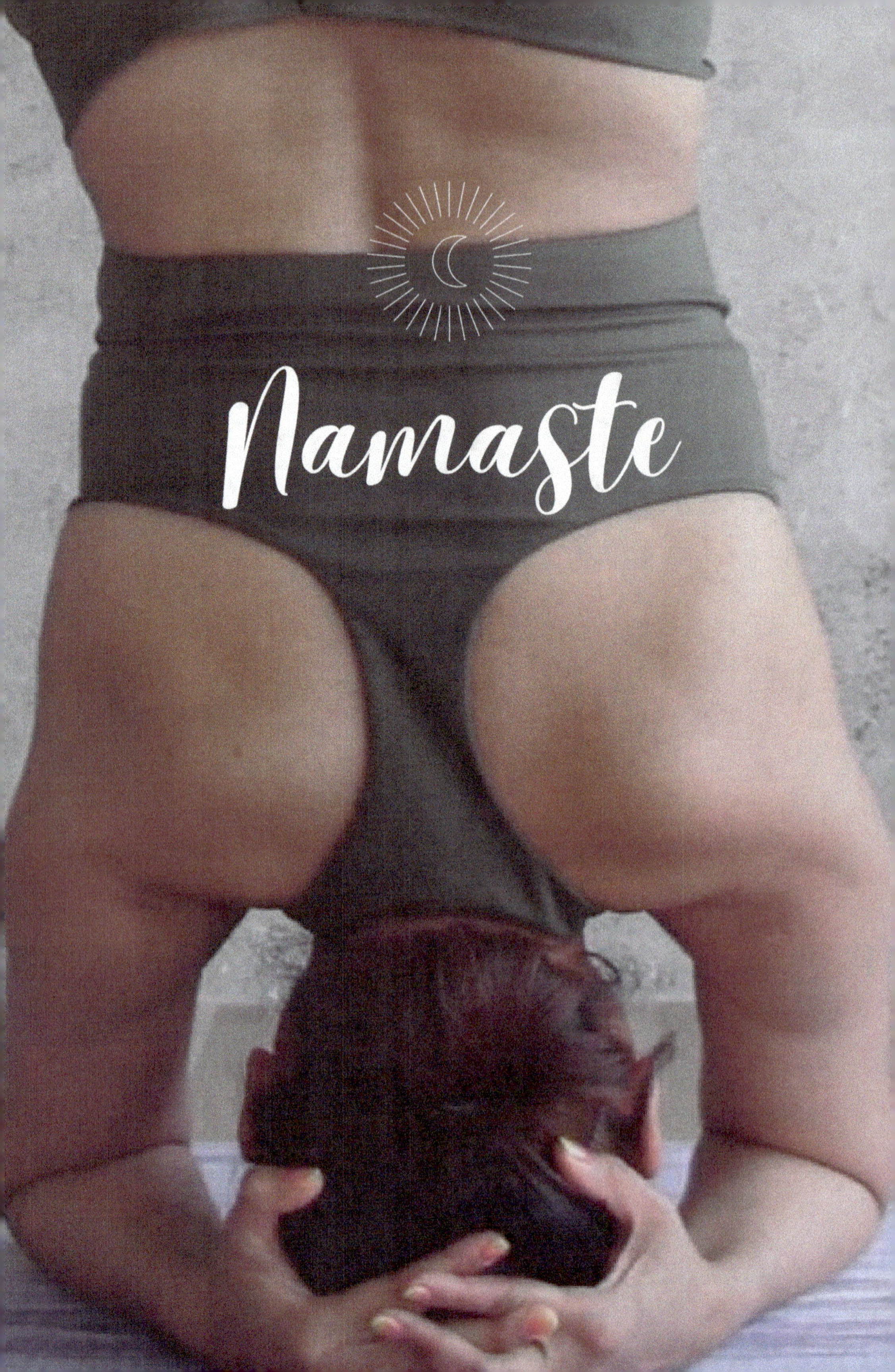
Namaste